The Bioethics of Pain Management

In this book, public health ethicist Daniel S. Goldberg sets out to characterize the subjective experience of pain and its undertreatment within the U.S. medical establishment, and puts forward public policy recommendations for ameliorating the undertreatment of pain. The book begins from the position that the overwhelming focus on opioid analgesics as a means for improving the undertreatment of pain is flawed, and argues instead that dominant Western models of biomedicine and objectivity delegitimize subjective knowledge of the body and pain in the U.S. This general intolerance for the subjectivity of pain is part of a specific American culture of pain in which a variety of actors take part, including not only physicians and health care providers, but also pain sufferers, caregivers, and policymakers. Concentrating primarily on bioethics, history, and public policy, the book brings a truly interdisciplinary approach to an urgent practical ethical problem. Taking up the practical challenge, the book culminates in a series of policy recommendations that provide pathways for moral agents to move beyond contests over drug policy to policy arenas that, based on the evidence, hold more promise in their capacity to address the devastating and inequitable undertreatment of pain in the U.S.

Daniel S. Goldberg is Assistant Professor in the Department of Bioethics and Interdisciplinary Studies in the Brody School of Medicine at East Carolina University, N.C.

Routledge Annals of Bioethics

Series Editors: Mark J. Cherry, St. Edward's University, USA,
Ana Smith Iltis, Saint Louis University, USA

The Bioethics of Pain Management

Beyond Opioids

Daniel S. Goldberg

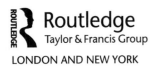

Routledge
Taylor & Francis Group

LONDON AND NEW YORK

First published 2014 by Routledge

2 Park Square, Milton Park, Abingdon, Oxfordshire OX14 4RN
711 Third Avenue, New York, NY 10017

*Routledge is an imprint of the Taylor & Francis Group,
an informa business*

First issued in paperback 2017

Library of Congress Cataloging-in-Publication Data

The bioethics of pain management : beyond opioids / edited by
Daniel S. Goldberg.
    pages cm. — (Routledge annals of bioethics ; 15)
    Includes bibliographical references and index.
    1. Chronic pain—Treatment—United States—Moral and ethical issues.
2. Opioids—Therapeutic use—Moral and ethical issues.   3. Opiod abuse—
United States.   4. Medical ethics.   I. Goldberg, Daniel S., 1977–
editor of compilation.
    RC483.5.O64B56 2014
    174.2'90472—dc23
    2013037045

ISBN. 978-0-415-74673-1 (hbk)
ISBN: 978-0-8153-7201-1 (pbk)

Typeset in Sabon
by Apex CoVantage, LLC

Contents

SECTION IV
Towards Ethical, Evidence-Based Pain Policy   95

Figures

Acknowledgements

This book could not have been completed without the patience, guidance, and understanding of a great many people. I would first like to thank all of my professors and colleagues at the Institute for the Medical Humanities in the University of Texas Medical Branch for creating an educational experience that has forever changed me. In particular, I would like to thank the members of my dissertation committee: Howard Brody, Melvyn Schreiber, Michele Carter, Jason Glenn, and Ben Rich for continually challenging me. Bill Winslade, the chair of my committee, has been my mentor, advisor, and confidant for almost 15 years. I cannot thank him enough, nor heap enough credit upon him for whatever I have managed to accomplish.

Special thanks go to the series editors for the *Annals of Bioethics*, Mark Cherry and Ana Iltis, for believing in the project and for their stewardship during the editing and review process.

I owe a great debt of gratitude to my colleagues in the Department of Bioethics & Interdisciplinary Studies at East Carolina University. Particular thanks is owed to Kenneth A. DeVille and Todd Savitt for shepherding me through the process of revising and improving this book.

I must thank my family of origin—Mom, Dad, Josh, Seth, and Zeide—for the honey on the pages of my books. To my wife Yuko Kishimoto, Ph.D., no words of gratitude are sufficient, only a life spent building a building. Finally, to my daughter Maya: may your ship sail far away from the shores of pain.

Preface

Emily Dickinson famously wrote that "[p]ain has an element of blank. . . ." Among several possible meanings, this phrase seems to imply that pain itself is nameless, that it defies categories, definitions, and even descriptions. Accordingly, as the subject of this book is the undertreatment of pain in American society, a number of questions immediately present themselves:

- Under what definition of pain am I operating?
- If different kinds of pain produce different experiences and different levels of treatment, which kinds of pain will I assess?
- How do the redemptive possibilities of pain factor into an assessment of its meaning?
- What is the relationship between pain and suffering?

Sketching out some responses to these questions will hopefully clarify the approach I am taking to understanding the undertreatment of pain in American society.

THE DEFINITION OF PAIN

The most widely used definition of pain is that provided by the International Association for the Study of Pain (IASP): "An unpleasant sensory and emotional experience associated with actual or potential tissue damage, or described in terms of such damage."[1] Yet, as many have noted, this definition is merely a starting point. Pain can unquestionably exist in the absence of tissue damage, which raises one of the central questions this book is intended to answer: why are so many pain experiences, in the absence of visible lesions, questioned, delegitimized, or rejected outright? Moreover, the IASP definition leaves unresolved the complicated relationship between pain and suffering. For example, does depression qualify as pain under the IASP definition? Is the grief experienced at the death of a child pain?

In her masterful 2005 essay on stigma and chronic pain, anthropologist Jean E. Jackson quotes no less than 10 different definitions of chronic pain from the clinical literature. She reasons that "the highly contested definition of pain itself is a major reason why defining chronic pain as symptoms that persist beyond expected healing time, although true, does not take one very far."[2]

In addition to these difficulties, pain is not monolithic. Different kinds of pain are qualitatively different in important ways, and produce different experiences for the pain sufferer, as well as prompting different responses related to treatment, stigma, and care. It is plausible to suggest that there is no meaning of pain, but only meanings of pain. These issues raise the question of whether a single definition of pain is coherent at all. If not, how is it even possible to talk of pain?

In prior work, I have adopted what I call a 'nonessentialist' approach to various questions related to health and illness in society.[3] Drawing largely on the work of later Wittgenstein, I have argued that we do not require an analytic definition of a word or a concept in order to use it meaningfully in practice.[4] In this book, I conceptualize pain from this vantage point, and thus I intentionally do not offer a definition of pain.

While the lack of such a definition does not preclude meaningful discussion of pain in American society, nothing in Wittgenstein's account implies that precision in analysis is either impossible or undesirable. Rather, the point is simply that the precision sought cannot rise to the level of a strict definition. Moreover, it is precisely because pain is multivalent—its "element of blank," in Dickinson's words—that it is important to specify the kinds of pain that are being discussed at any particular level of analysis.

WHICH PAIN?

Clinical pain is typically designated as acute or chronic, though there are obviously many more categories applicable to different pain experiences. However, aside from many "problematic" kinds of chronic pain, the idea that most kinds of pain are treated well is unsupportable based on the best evidence. For example, as will be documented in Chapter 1, despite decades of efforts and the increasing visibility and availability of a clinical subspecialty devoted entirely to palliation, there is good evidence that persons suffering from acute pain secondary to terminal illness continue to receive inadequate treatment for their pain. Even the acknowledgment that many kinds of chronic pain present the most serious difficulties in clinical practice, ethics, and policy does not justify ignoring the evidence that many different kinds of pain sufferers do not receive sufficient treatment for their pain. The facts also show that in the vast majority of cases, safe and effective modalities exist for treating pain.

As such, this book's examination of the general undertreatment of pain in the U.S. precludes a specific focus on any one kind of pain. In addition, leaving pain as ambiguous and as multifaceted as it seems to exist in people's actual experiences is consistent with the phenomenological approach that I adopt as to pain, which will be explored in detail in Chapter 2. As Dickinson suggests, pain as a lived experience defies categories, straddles boundaries, and obliterates definitions. Accordingly, distinctions between different kinds of pain are at best useful heuristics, but are unavoidably crude. Finally, where there exist a number of safe and effective interventions for treating the overwhelming majority of pain experiences, it is difficult to perceive any meaningful ethical distinction that turns on whether the pain identified is chronic low back pain or acute pain secondary to mechanical trauma.[5]

Thus, this book does not focus on any one kind of pain experience in assessing the undertreatment of pain in American society. Although this choice undoubtedly introduces complexity into the analysis, I will argue that an interdisciplinary health humanities approach is particularly well-suited to making sense of such complexity.[6] Such an approach, which begins by acknowledging the interactions, complexities, and ambiguities of the phenomena of pain in society, is more promising as a means of making sense of the undertreatment of pain. There is little sense in ignoring the ambiguity, complexity, and multivalence of how people experience pain in the U.S., and an approach that welcomes such features as a way of thinking about the meaning of pain and its undertreatment can at least be assured of avoiding crude oversimplifications and resulting piecemeal policy solutions. Pain does indeed have an element of blank.

That said, as indicated above, precision is important. If I do not expressly focus on any single kind of pain, it is necessary to specify which type of pain is relevant to any particular point. There are reasons why chronic pain sufferers generally fare worse in seeking treatment than acute pain sufferers, and these reasons are crucial in producing policies that may ameliorate the undertreatment of pain. Some aspects of the analysis will be more applicable to some kinds of pain than others, and where this is so, I will specify as such and explain *why* it is so.

THE REDEMPTIVE POSSIBILITIES OF PAIN

One of the most intriguing questions about pain is whether it is, as some have suggested, "the worst of all evils,"[7] or whether the possibility of redemption through pain implies that pain may be a good of some sort. The literature on this question alone is immense and is a particularly rich vein of inquiry for all manner of social and cultural studies.

I do not discount the potential or the power of the narrative of redemption in giving meaning to experiences of pain; such a story has roots in the Judeo-Christian tradition as old as the Book of Job and is related in myriad ways in many other traditions.[8] However, the possibilities of redemption in pain are not the subject of this book. If a narrative of redemption aids illness sufferers in making meaning of their pain, that is all to the good. But there is an unavoidably pragmatic element to my project: there is general consensus that millions of Americans experience intense, sometimes incapacitating pain that may last for days and recur for years, and that many of these people do not receive available treatment that could significantly alleviate their suffering. I do not doubt that some of these sufferers' broken stories could be and are fixed through a narrative of redemption.[9] However, I deem it safe to suggest that whatever the power of such a narrative, it neither explains why so many experience pain when effective treatments exist nor necessarily offers succor to any particular pain sufferer.[10]

Similarly, Elaine Scarry, whose work has inspired a generation of pain scholars, notes her concern regarding

> a view that might seem to license the infliction of pain . . . On the one hand, we have to remember how a shaman can willfully take on pain and actually bring about amazing world-transforming effects through his own meditation on it. On the other hand, there is the kind of pain that a person has no say over, did not authorize, and does not have the option of expressing in . . . beautiful language.[11]

Moreover, she observes, even acknowledging the "vast tonal and thematic differences," talk of the redemptive possibilities of pain "from the medical world" could be perceived by the sufferer as "a horribly crude way of saying: 'It's okay that you're in pain. There is great meaning to be built from this, so live with it.'"[12]

Similarly, many ethnographies of pain sufferers reveal that narratives of redemption are frequently either absent or are regarded as inadequate as a means of making meaning of the sufferers' pain. Not all pain sufferers are optimistic and hopeful; some are embittered and broken.[13] In my view, not even the most ardent proponent of the redemptive qualities of pain is justified in suggesting that such qualities are a sufficient answer to the question of why so many Americans suffer so much pain for which safe and effective treatments exist.

PAIN AND SUFFERING

Most experts agree that pain and suffering are distinguishable. If so, it is possible to suffer without pain or to experience pain without suffering. However, trying to explain the relationship between pain and suffering is extraordinarily difficult. To return to an earlier example, it seems difficult to deny that depression produces suffering in some sense, but it does not necessarily follow that depression produces pain. To argue that depression causes mental but not physical pain is obviously circular and sheds no light on the issue of what, if anything, distinguishes physical from mental pain. Such a response also seems to assume the coherence of some kind of mind-body duality, which, I shall argue in Chapter 5, is a primary factor in the under-treatment of pain in the U.S.

Of course, in many pain experiences the subject does indeed suffer. Some have argued for a distinction between kinds of pain that centers on the purpose of the pain. Some kinds of pain "serve an important biological (or evolutionary) function in that it warns the organism of impending danger, informs the organism of tissue damage or injury, or deters the organism from interfering with healing or causing further tissue damage."[14] Thus, an entirely painless existence turns out to cause a number of serious health problems. Known as congenital analgesia, individuals who have this rare genetic disorder often suffer repeated injury, including broken bones, lacerated skin, and damage to internal body tissues, resulting in significantly shortened life expectancy.[15]

Other kinds of pain, such as chronic pain that persists for years without relief or explanation, seem to serve no identifiable "biological" purpose, and hence may be more likely to cause distinct kinds of suffering. Even "useful" pain may cause suffering, but it may in truth be easier to make meaning out of "useful" pain than pain which seems "purposeless."

In any case, this project does not aim to disentangle the pain from suffering. With good evidentiary support, I take it as a given that many kinds of pain experiences produce kinds of suffering, even acknowledging that different pain experiences likely produce different kinds and intensities of suffering. Like many of the other choices I make in conceptualizing the undertreatment of pain, leaving the relationship between pain and suffering as ambiguous, as complicated, and as multivalent as it seems to be in people's lived experiences embodies the phenomenologic approach to pain adopted in this book. Moreover, because of the nonessentialist approach I take to pain, such ambiguity does not preclude meaningful thought about pain and suffering, nor does it undermine my pragmatic goal: the production of policies that justify the hope that the undertreatment of pain in the U.S. will be ameliorated.

TERMINOLOGY

Finally, I offer here an explanation of the term I will use to refer to the subject in pain: the *pain sufferer*. This is simply a variant of the phrase *illness sufferer*, which is widely used in the health humanities. The notion of an illness sufferer is both broader and more accurate than the clinical term *patient*, because while illness sufferers may often be patients over the duration of any given illness experience, there are also likely to be many moments where they are not actively patients.

Terming the subject in pain a *pain sufferer* may seem to beg the question regarding the connection between pain and suffering. As noted above, I am content to leave the relationship complex and ambiguous and do not, by referring to the subject in pain as a *pain sufferer* mean to suggest that pain necessarily requires suffering. It is a basic precept of the health humanities that the human experiences of illness and pain are limited only by the boundless capacity of the human search for meaning. Just as referring to the person undergoing an illness experience as the *illness sufferer* does not negate the immense variety of experiences in the face of illness, speaking of the subject in pain as the *pain sufferer* does not commit me to any firm position on the extent, if any, to which the person in pain suffers. Given how vast and deep the undertreatment of pain goes in the U.S. (documented in Section I), it seems safe to suggest that large numbers of persons in pain do in fact suffer.

NOTES

1. International Association for the Study of Pain, *Pain Definitions: Pain*, accessed March 16, 2008, from http://www.iasp-pain.org/AM/Template.cfm?Section=General_Resource_Links&Template=/CM/HTMLDisplay.cfm&ContentID=3058#Pain

2. Jean E. Jackson, "Stigma, Liminality, and Chronic Pain: Mind-Body Borderlands," *American Ethnologist* 32, no. 3 (August 2005): 335.

3. Daniel S. Goldberg, "Religion, the Culture of Biomedicine, and the Tremendum: Towards a Non-Essentialist Analysis of Interconnection," *Journal of Religion and Health* 46, no. 1 (March 2007): 99–108.

4. Daniel S. Goldberg, "Eschewing Definitions of the Therapeutic Misconception: A Family Resemblance Analysis," *Journal of Medicine & Philosophy* 36, no. 3 (2011): 296–320; Sorin Bangu, "Later Wittgenstein on Essentialism, Family Resemblance and Philosophical Method," *Metaphysica* 6, no. 2 (2005): 53–73; and Marie McGinn, *Wittgenstein and the Philosophical Investigations* (London, UK: Routledge Press, 1997).

5. However, this is *not* to claim that there are no meaningful distinctions between different kinds of pain. As I have expressly argued, different kinds of pain produce different phenomenologies of pain. The argument here is that the ethics of the body in pain do not turn on a precise demarcation between types of pain.

6. William H. Newell, "A Theory of Interdisciplinary Studies," *Issues in Integrative Studies* 19 (2001): 1–25.

7. Thomas H. Dormandy, *The Worst of Evils: The Fight against Pain* (New Haven, CT: Yale University Press, 2006).

8. Luis O. Gomez, "Pain and the Suffering Consciousness: The Alleviation of Suffering in Buddhist Discourse," in *Pain and Its Transformations: The Interface of Biology and Culture*, eds. Sarah Coakley and Kay Kaufman Shelemay (Cambridge, MA: Harvard University Press, 2007), 101–21; Elizabeth Tolbert, "Voice, Metaphysics, and Community: Pain and Transformation in the Finnish-Karelian Ritual Lament," in *Pain and Its Transformations: The Interface of Biology and Culture*, eds. Sarah Coakley and Kay Kaufman Shelemay (Cambridge, MA: Harvard University Press, 2007), 147–65; and Martha Ann Selby, "The Poetics of Anesthesia: Representations of Pain in the Literatures of Classical India," in *Pain and Its Transformations: The Interface of Biology and Culture*, eds. Sarah Coakley and Kay Kaufman Shelemay (Cambridge, MA: Harvard University Press, 2007), 317–30.

9. Howard A. Brody, *Stories of Sickness* (New Haven, CT: Yale University Press, 1987).

10. Jean E. Jackson, "How to Narrate Pain? The Politics of Representation," in *Narrative, Pain, and Suffering*, eds. Daniel B. Carr, John David Loeser, and David B. Morris (Seattle, WA: IASP Press, 2003), 230–42.

11. Elaine Scarry and Arthur Kleinman, "Reductionism and the Separation of 'Suffering' and 'Pain,'" in *Pain and Its Transformations: The Interface of Biology and Culture*, eds. Sarah Coakley and Kay Kaufman Shelemay (Cambridge, MA: Harvard University Press, 2007), 139.

12. Ibid.

13. Sandra P. Thomas and Mary Johnson, "A Phenomenologic Study of Chronic Pain," *Western Journal of Nursing Research* 22, no. 6 (October 2000): 683–705.

14. David B. Resnik, Marsha Rehm, and Raymond B. Minard, "The Undertreatment of Pain: Scientific, Clinical, Cultural, and Philosophical Factors," *Medicine, Health Care and Philosophy* 4, no. 3 (October 2001): 280.

15. Niranjan Biswal, Murali Sundaram, Betsy Mathai, and Sijay Balasubramanian, "Congenital Indifference to Pain," *Indian Journal of Pediatrics* 65, no. 5 (September 1998): 755–69; Eric Hirsch, Danny Moye, and Joseph H. Dimon III, "Congenital Indifference to Pain: Long-term Follow-up of Two Cases," *Southern Medical Journal* 88, no. 8 (August 1995): 851–57.

Introduction
The Power of the Visible and the Undertreatment of Pain in the U.S.

"That which is not on the scale of the gaze falls outside the domain of possible knowledge."[1]
—Michel Foucault, *The Birth of the Clinic*

Two questions animate this project:

1. Given that the vast majority of pain experiences can be adequately managed using available treatment modalities, why does pain remain so poorly treated in the U.S.?
2. Given the immense and crossdisciplinary scholarship, advocacy, and policy attention directed to the undertreatment of pain in the U.S., why does pain remain so poorly treated?

As to the first question, the failure to treat pain adequately in the U.S. cannot be attributed to a lack of safe and effective treatments. An overwhelming majority of pain experiences can be alleviated using currently available interventions.[2] This fact suggests that the reasons for the undertreatment of pain go far beyond any analysis of the clinical efficacies of various interventions. This does not imply that such interventions are unimportant. Attitudes and beliefs towards, for example, opioid analgesics and addiction are relevant to the undertreatment of pain. However, these attitudes and beliefs cannot be separated from an analysis of how individuals and communities conceive of pain itself. Medicines are social "objects" in the sense that their meaning is necessarily shaped by social, cultural, and contextual factors.[3] Thus, any analysis of the undertreatment of pain that focuses merely on specific remedies for treating pain without consideration of the social and cultural contexts in which pain is interpreted and understood is incomplete.[4]

As to the second question, the failure to treat pain adequately has not gone unnoticed in the U.S. There is an immense literature on the undertreatment of pain across and beyond medicine and clinical practice to biomedical research, ethics, health policy, sociology, anthropology, history, public health, nursing, social work, disability studies, literature, psychology, communications, etc. The problem has sparked a storm of attention, with scores of articles, books, and policy analyses available, funding opportunities across public, private, and nonprofit sectors, focus from multiple professional societies, and the energies of numerous community-based organizations and advocacy efforts related to pain.

Despite nearly three decades of such attention, there is little evidence that pain is generally being treated better, and even less evidence of improvement in treating chronic pain.[5] Moreover, as the number of chronically ill and disabled persons increases,[6] there is every reason to suspect that the prevalence and incidence of pain will also increase. In addition, inequalities in the diagnosis and treatment of pain are significant and are widening.[7]

If the undertreatment of pain has been relatively common knowledge for decades and if the problem has enjoyed no lack of attention, why is it that pain remains so poorly treated in the U.S.? This is one question this book is intended to address. An additional question is what are the limitations of current ethics and policy approaches to the undertreatment of pain? Ultimately, if it is ethically important to treat pain, it is critical to ascertain exactly why prevailing approaches do not seem to be effective in improving the treatment of pain.

This book has three main objectives: First, it aims to explain why a social and cultural analysis of pain in the U.S. is a prerequisite to understanding the undertreatment of pain and to proposing workable solutions. Second, it uses this analysis to explain why prevailing approaches have not alleviated the undertreatment of pain and are unlikely to do so. Third, it produces policy recommendations based on the social and cultural analysis of pain in context of American society. These policy recommendations reflect the best evidence regarding the causes of the undertreatment of pain, and therefore justify hope that their implementation could ameliorate such undertreatment.

This book's commitment to evidence-based policy requires engaging the ongoing debate over the meaning and validity of the terms "evidence-based policy" and "evidence-based medicine." Many criticisms of evidence-based medicine attack the cramped view of what qualifies as relevant evidence. Thus, numerous commentators have pointed out the problems of relying on the evidence produced from randomized controlled trials (RCTs) as the so-called 'gold standard' regardless of the subject being studied.[8] Depending on the nature of the question to be answered, other kinds of evidence and analytical modalities may be vastly superior to the RCT.

For example, few would suggest that the best means of gaining insight into what it *feels* like for a person to live with chronic pain is via an RCT. As a form of knowledge production, the RCT aims to strip away individual variations in the hopes of maintaining high internal validity.[9] In contrast, the entire point of an inquiry into the lived experiences of the chronic pain sufferer is to learn something about those *individual* experiences. Not coincidentally, the vast majority of studies devoted to assessing the lived experiences of chronic pain employ narrative, phenomenologic, and related qualitative approaches.[10] These approaches aim to center the subject in pain, which is a central theme of this book.

SECTION I: THE LIVED EXPERIENCE OF PAIN

Because centering the subject in pain is paramount, Section I addresses the lived experience of pain. The basic idea is that the pain sufferers' lived experiences are generally not centered in biomedical encounters in which relief for pain is sought. Accordingly, in Chapter 1 (this volume), I survey the evidence relating to the epidemiology of pain so as to provide a basic understanding of the prevalence and distribution of pain within and between different populations and communities in the U.S. This approach contextualizes the subject of Chapter 2 (this volume), which addresses the phenomenology of pain—that is, what it is like to "be-in-the-world" as a pain sufferer.[11]

SECTION II: HISTORY, THE POWER OF THE VISIBLE, AND PAIN

Once I have articulated an account of the epidemiology and phenomenology of pain in Section I, Section II explains why the lived experiences of the pain sufferer are generally not privileged. This explanation will focus on an account of how pain came to mean what it has come to mean in American culture. My argument is that because traditionally dominant policy approaches to improving the undertreatment of pain have taken little account of either what pain currently means or, perhaps more importantly, what social and cultural factors combined to produce those meanings, they have not been and are unlikely to be successful in reducing the needless suffering of millions of Americans. From Section I's focus on the lived experience of pain, Section II reaches back chronologically and conceptually to assess the social and cultural power of the visible lesion in biomedical culture.

The visible lesion is particularly relevant to thinking about pain because pain is generally taken to be an invisible, subjective phenomenon. Pain is problematic in American culture because it cannot be seen in the body, and this problem is a prime factor in its undertreatment. Chapter 3 (this volume) traces the connection between pain and the need for visible lesions to explain it in the nineteenth century and introduces one of the major theoretical frameworks upon which this project rests: Michel Foucault's analysis of the rise of the "clinical gaze." Because medical perception is front and center in Foucault's analysis, his framework is especially well-suited for a project devoted to tracing the impact of the visible lesion in American cultures of biomedicine and science.

Chapter 3 (this volume) brings this lens to bear on the problem of pain without lesion in mid- to late nineteenth-century America. The central question here is as the anatomoclinical method took hold during the nineteenth century, how did physicians account for pain that could not be connected with any material pathology or lesion inside the body? Answering this question is integral to comprehending the role visible pathology plays in the contemporary undertreatment of pain, and therefore Chapter 3 (this volume) utilizes a number of neurological and medical primary sources to ground an argument that pain without lesion was not tenable to leading lights of American medicine.

Foucault does not expressly connect his work on medical perception to the contemporary treatment of pain. However, one of the most influential pain scholars of the last few decades, David B. Morris, has picked up the theme and argues that Foucault's analysis can explain how it is that pain came to be seen as "invisible" in the West during the nineteenth century.[12] Morris's arguments have come under fire from multiple authorities on the history of pain.[13]

Accordingly, a key objective in Chapter 3 (this volume) is to fill some of the evidentiary gaps in Morris's argument. But more than simply filling gaps, I argue that many of the criticisms of Morris's argument are based on a misinterpretation. Morris does not claim that nineteenth-century physicians ignored or trivialized their patients' pain. Chapter 3 (this volume) shows that while nineteenth-century physicians did not typically invalidate their patients' pain—or at least their socially privileged patients' pain—but nevertheless, in an important sense pain in the absence of visible, material pathology vanished from medical (and cultural) perception. After articulating this thesis, I explain in Chapter 4 (this volume) how these mid- to late nineteenth-century attitudes towards pain without lesion have profound implications for the contemporary undertreatment of pain in the U.S. Some of the roots of the undertreatment of pain can be found in these nineteenth-century attitudes, practices, and beliefs.

In addition, Chapter 4 (this volume) picks up the evidence surveyed in chapters 2 and 3 (this volume), suggesting that conceptions of the relationship between mind and body play a crucial role in shaping and informing the meaning of pain in American culture. Part of the problem in the common distinction drawn between "mental" and "physical" pain is that it reinforces a deeply flawed concept of mind-body dualism that pervades understandings of pain.[14] This is problematic because adherence to mind-body dualism is a major factor in the undertreatment of pain, and also plays a significant role in producing the stigma that pain sufferers so frequently endure.[15]

SECTION III: ETHICS, SUBJECTIVITY, AND PAIN

Chapter 5 (this volume) connects this adherence to such dualism and to the power of the visible lesion via analysis of functional magnetic resonance imaging (fMRI) techniques. By measuring blood oxygenation levels in precise areas of the brain that are known to be associated with pain, fMRI techniques have enabled investigators to identify neural correlates of pain.[16] Many of these studies have either implied or stated that fMRI techniques have finally provided objective evidence of pain.[17] There is, however, evidence that both scientists and the mass media may overstate the meaning and significance of fMRI studies.[18]

Although evaluating the claims of fMRI proponents as to pain is important, it is also necessary to ask why producing objective evidence of pain matters? Why are these claims socially, culturally, and clinically significant? Accordingly, Chapter 5 (this volume) addresses these questions by analyzing some of the philosophical and neuroscientific debates over the significance of subjectivity in concepts of consciousness and pain.

It is no accident that philosophers and neuroscientists alike frequently refer to pain in their discourses on consciousness: pain is a paradigm case of consciousness. Insofar as the role of subjectivity in consciousness has important implications for the ways pain and the relation between the mind and the body is conceived in American culture, any account of social and cultural beliefs and practices about pain must assess cultural narratives and perspectives on consciousness, subjectivity, and pain. These meanings overlap in substantial ways with the meaning of fMRI studies of pain. Chapter 5 (this volume) assesses these issues in context of ethics, subjectivity, and pain.

In Chapter 6 (this volume), I continue the analysis developed in Chapter 5 (this volume) related to the general cultural distaste for subjective ways of knowing in context of health, illness, and pain, and I examine the effect this preference has in American bioethics. I survey the conceptual work that moral objectivism does in its most dominant form within bioethics discourse—principlism—and explain why principlism in its prevailing forms is inadequate for a rich and informed notion of the ethics of pain. In its place, I extend the discussion in Chapter 2 (this volume) centered on the phenomenology of pain and address its ethical implications.

SECTION IV: TOWARDS ETHICAL, EVIDENCE-BASED PAIN POLICY

The move to ethical, evidence-based pain policies is the subject of Section IV, which is comprised of the final two chapters. For many reasons, I eschew an approach that tracks the general emphasis within pain policy and ethics on opioids and the opioid regulatory scheme.

The currently prevailing approach to the undertreatment of pain focuses on the need for balance in pain policy.[19] Balance is sought between the need to prevent diversion of opioid analgesics for illegal purposes and the need to use such analgesics in treating pain sufferers. There is of course nothing inherently wrong with the goal of balance in pain policy. Who would endorse unbalanced public policy of any kind?

However, one flaw with this approach is that regulatory schemes are themselves social phenomena that are animated by a host of political, social, and cultural beliefs, attitudes, and practices.[20] However well-intentioned, simply tweaking the regulatory scheme sheds no light on why the scheme is unbalanced to begin with. If the goal is to create policy that encourages the proper use of appropriate medications for the treatment of pain, it is necessary to address the root social causes that drive unbalanced pain policy.

Moreover, focusing almost exclusively on opioid regulation leaves obscure the effect of social and cultural beliefs and attitudes towards pain itself. There is little doubt that these beliefs and attitudes influence the treatment of pain. To take just one example, there is good evidence that elderly populations significantly underreport their pain.[21] Given that the health-care provider's primary means of assessing pain is through the patient's self-report, a patient's unwillingness to report his/her own pain is a significant impediment to effective treatment of pain. Yet it is unclear how addressing the regulatory scheme for opioid distribution will do anything to ameliorate this problem. Indeed, it is not apparent how the prevailing policy approach even accounts for such a problem.

Nevertheless, while I do not share the belief that improving the opioid regulatory scheme is likely to substantially improve the undertreatment of pain in the U.S., it is undeniable that opioid policy is relevant. Therefore, in Chapter 7 (this volume), I touch on some of the debate over opioids, both to explain what I do (and do not) think is important about that debate and to justify an approach that does not dwell on such interventions.

Tracking my approach that deemphasizes the significance for opioid policy in thinking about the undertreatment of pain in the U.S., I similarly avoid focusing on the connection between fears of addiction and the undertreatment of pain. As I am expressly arguing that the undue focus on opioids has not improved the undertreatment of pain, it follows that a similar focus on alleviating the fears of addiction to opioids is unlikely to result in significant improvement. As with opioids in general, I agree the issue of addiction is relevant, and I will mention it in Chapter 7 (this volume). Nevertheless, while the issue of addiction certainly merits deep analysis on its own terms, I argue that it is not of central importance in explaining the undertreatment of pain.

The obvious objection here is that, even assuming the criticisms of the general focus on opioids within pain policy and ethics has merit, it remains unclear why and how an interdisciplinary health humanities approach promises to improve on currently dominant approaches. The short answer is that enhanced understanding of the social and cultural roots of our practices and attitudes towards pain will facilitate the creation of policy recommendations that may justify some measure of confidence in their capacity for improving the undertreatment of pain.

A slightly longer answer requires reference to the medieval and Renaissance humanists from whom we derive the educational program known as the humanities.[22] One of the key tenets of the humanist ethos was an emphasis on practical engagement. That is, the Renaissance humanists expressly rejected the earlier Scholastic tendency to bandy abstractions that had little relevance for people's daily lives and that did even less to encourage virtue.[23]

Utilizing scholarship as a means of producing knowledge that is informed by and relevant to our actual practices is a core precept of the humanities. Therefore, in an important sense, the humanists were early translational researchers. While a social and cultural analysis of the meaning of pain in American society is hopefully a worthy contribution in its own right, if such an analysis is unmoored from an attempt to translate such theory into practice, it is arguably inconsistent with the ethos of the humanists. A project more faithful to the lessons of the humanists must translate its social and cultural "evidence" into policy recommendations intended to produce practical changes in relevant actors' actual practices.

Chapter 8 (this volume) assimilates all of the arguments and analyses developed in the first seven chapters into three separate policies intended to address the undertreatment of pain in the U.S. These policies attend to the deeply rooted social and cultural forces that shape the meaning of pain in American society, and then bring this attention to the level of the pain sufferer him- or herself. The recommended pain policies are specifically directed to the actors who enjoy the capacity to change the relevant behaviors. The intended policy audiences include federal and state regulators, professional health administrators, professional health educators, and pain policy scholars, as well as pain advocates, caregivers, and pain sufferers themselves.

As suggested above, constructing a useful notion of evidence-based policy requires an understanding of the evidence as to pain that is both deeper and broader than is generally conceived of and utilized in both evidence-based medicine and evidence-based health policy. This book is devoted to the production and synthesis of evidence in the larger sense of the term, evidence that includes analysis of the social and cultural beliefs, attitudes, and practices regarding the meaning of pain. These "variables" are prime determinants in the undertreatment of pain. This sociocultural evidence base is incorporated in the policy recommendations detailed in Chapter 8 (this volume), which is why I term them "evidence-based policy recommendations."

The tension between the broader and narrower senses of the evidence base that ought to be used in constructing pain policies is not semantics. The statistics regarding the prevalence of pain and the failures in treating it are staggering, as Chapter 1 (this volume) document. If policies intended to improve these problems are unlikely to be successful because they fail to consider the social and cultural factors that animate the undertreatment of pain, then opportunities to reduce the suffering of millions of people may be lost or undermined.

In part, my argument is that a thorough comprehension of the myriad ways in which attitudes and beliefs about pain shape the treatment of pain may dispel the notion that focusing simply on opioid regulation is sufficient to alleviate the suffering of the millions of Americans who endure pain without adequate treatment. I turn now to Chapter 1 (this volume) in the hopes of documenting the scope of their suffering.

NOTES

1. Michel Foucault, *The Birth of the Clinic: An Archaeology of Medical Perception*, trans. Alan M. Sheridan Smith (New York, NY: Vintage Books, 1994), 166.
2. Noting that the majority of pain experiences can be ameliorated is an oversimplification, of course, because different pain experiences are more or less susceptible to different interventions. I will address this issue in more detail in Chapter 1 and Chapter 8 (this volume).
3. Joseph Gabriel, "Gods and Monsters: Drugs, Addiction, and the Origins of Narcotic Control in the 19th Century Urban North" (PhD dissertation, Rutgers University, 2006); Susan Reynolds Whyte, Sjakk van der Geest, and Anita Hardon, *The Social Lives of Medicines* (Cambridge, UK: Cambridge University Press, 2002); and Bruno Latour, *We Have Never Been Modern* (Cambridge, MA: Harvard University Press, 1993).
4. Gabriel, "Gods and Monsters"; Caroline Jean Acker, *Creating the American Junkie: Addiction Research in the Classic Era of Narcotic Control* (Baltimore, MD: Johns Hopkins University Press, 2002); Caroline Jean Acker, "From All Purposes Anodyne to Marker of Deviance: Physicians' Attitudes towards Opioids in the US from 1890 to 1940," in *Drugs and Narcotics in History*, eds. Roy Porter and Mikulas Teich (Cambridge, UK: Cambridge University Press, 1995), 114–32.
5. Noémi R. Tousignant, "Pain and the Pursuit of Objectivity: Pain-Measuring Technologies in the United States c. 1890–1975" (Ph.D. dissertation, McGill University, 2006). I will address in detail the empirical evidence regarding the prevalence, incidence, and undertreatment of pain in Chapter 1 (this volume).
6. Ross DeVol and Armen Bedroussian, *An Unhealthy America: The Economic Burden of Chronic Disease* (Santa Monica, CA: Milken Institute, 2007).
7. See Lisa J. Staton, Mukta Panda, Ian Chen, Inginia Genao, James Kurz, Mark Pasanen, Alex J. Mechaber, Madhusudan Menon, Jane O'Rorke, JoAnn Wood, Eric Rosenberg, Charles Faeslis, Tim Carey, Diane Calleson, and Sam Cykert, "When Race Matters: Disagreement in Pain Perception between Patients and Their Physicians in Primary Care," *Journal of the National Medical Association* 99, no. 5 (May 2007): 532–37; Carmen R. Green, Karen O. Anderson, Tamara A. Baker, Lisa C. Campbell, Sheila Decker, Roger B. Fillingim, Donna A. Kaloukalani, Kathyrn E. Lasch, Cynthia Myers, Raymond C. Tait, Knox H. Todd, and April H. Vallerand, "The Unequal Burden of Pain: Confronting Racial and Ethnic Disparities in Pain," *Pain Medicine* 4, no. 3 (September 2003): 277–94.
8. Jason Grossman, "A Couple of the Nasties Lurking in Evidence-Based Medicine," *Social Epistemology* 22, no. 4 (October 2008): 333–52; Adam La Caze, "Evidence-Based Medicine Can't Be . . . ," *Social Epistemology* 22, no. 4 (October 2008): 353–70; Howard Brody, Franklin G. Miller, and Elizabeth Bogdan-Lovis, "Evidence-Based Medicine: Watching out for Its Friends,"

Perspectives in Biology and Medicine 48, no. 4 (Autumn 2005): 570–84; Ross G. Upshur, "Looking for Rules in a World of Exceptions: Reflections on Evidence-Based Practice," *Perspectives on Biology and Medicine* 48, no. 4 (Autumn 2005): 477–89.

9. Indeed, Noémi Tousignant documents this phenomenon in context of Henry Beecher's pioneering work on analgesic clinical trials, which showed that clinically useful information about pain was best produced by aggregating individual experiences into a larger distribution. Tousignant, "Pain and the Pursuit of Objectivity"; Noémi Tousignant, "The Rise and Fall of the Dolorimeter: Pain, Analgesics, and the Management of Subjectivity in Mid-twentieth-Century United States," *Journal of the History of Medicine and Allied Sciences* 66, no. 2 (2010): 145–79.

10. See, e.g., Jackson, "Stigma, Liminality, and Chronic Pain"; Jean E. Jackson, *Camp Pain: Talking with Chronic Pain Patients* (Philadelphia, PA: University of Pennsylvania Press, 2000); Jean E. Jackson, "'After a While No One Believes You': Real and Unreal Pain," in *Pain as Human Experience*, eds. Paul E. Brodwin, Arthur Kleinman, Byron J. Good, and Mary-Jo DelVecchio Good (Berkeley, CA: University of California Press), 138–68; Marja-Liisa Honkasalo, "Chronic Pain as a Posture towards the World," *Scandinavian Journal of Psychology* 41, no. 3 (September 2000): 197–208; Marja-Liisa Honkasalo, "What Is Chronic Is Ambiguity: Encountering Biomedicine with Long-Lasting Pain," *Journal of the Finnish Anthropological Society* 24, no. 4 (1999): 75–92; Thomas and Johnson, "A Phenomenologic Study of Chronic Pain."

11. The interplay between the population-based approach of Chapter 1 (this volume) and the phenomenologic focus of Chapter 2 (this volume) itself characterizes some key aspects of the medical humanities analysis I will use here. My general aim is to unpack some of the social and cultural meanings of pain in the United States and then apply these understandings to assess and center the lived subject in pain. This tacking back and forth between larger social representations and narratives and the subject's lived experiences of pain within their particular communities and networks is part of what an interdisciplinary medical humanities approach can offer.

12. David B. Morris, "An Invisible History of Pain: Early 19th-Century Britain and America," *Clinical Journal of Pain* 14, no. 3 (September 1998): 191–96; and David B. Morris, *The Culture of Pain* (Berkeley, CA: University of California Press, 1991).

13. Andrew Hodgkiss, *From Lesion to Metaphor: Chronic Pain in British, French, and German Medical Writings 1800–1914* (Amsterdam, Netherlands: Rodopi Press, 2000).

14. Jackson, "Stigma, Liminality, and Chronic Pain"; and John Searle, *The Rediscovery of Mind* (Cambridge, MA: The MIT Press, 1992).

15. Jackson, "Stigma, Liminality, and Chronic Pain"; and Jackson, *Camp Pain*.

16. The term *correlate* is important and has been the source of much confusion, which I will address in Chapter 5 (this volume).

17. Thorsten Giesecke, Richard H. Gracely, Masilo A.B. Grant, Alf Nachemson, Frank Petzke, David A. Williams, and Daniel J. Clauw, "Evidence of Augmented Central Pain Processing in Idiopathic Chronic Low Back Pain," *Arthritis & Rheumatism* 50, no. 2 (February 2004): 613–623; and Robert C. Coghill, John G. McHaffie, and Ye-Fen Yen, "Neural Correlates of Interindividual Differences in the Subjective Experience of Pain," *Proceedings in the National Academy of Sciences* 100, no. 14 (July 8, 2003): 8538–42.

18. Edward Vul, Christine Harris, Piotr Winkielman, and Harold Pashler, "Puzzlingly High Correlations in fMRI Studies of Emotion, Personality, and

Social Cognition," *Perspectives in Psychological Science* 4, no. 3 (April 2009): 274–90; Michael S. Pardo and Dennis Patterson, "Philosophical Foundations of Law and Neuroscience," *University of Illinois Law Review* 2010, no. 4 (2010): 1211–50; and Amanda Pustilnik, "Violence on the Brain: A Critique of Neuroscience in Criminal Law," *Wake Forest Law Review* 44 (2009): 183–237.

19. Aaron M. Gilson, David E. Joranson, Karen M. Ryan, Martha A. Maurer, Jody P. Moen, and Janet F. Kline, *Achieving Balance in Federal and State Pain Policy* (Madison, WI: Pain & Policy Studies Group, University of Wisconsin Paul B. Carbone Comprehensive Cancer Center, 2008), accessed June 3, 2009, from http://www.painpolicy.wisc.edu/Achieving_Balance/index.html.

20. Shai Joshua Lavi, *The Modern Art of Dying: Euthanasia in the United States* (Princeton, NJ: Princeton University Press, 2006).

21. Daniel S. Goldberg, "The Sole Indexicality of Pain: How Attitudes towards the Elderly Erect Barriers to Pain Management," *Michigan State University Journal of Medicine & Law* 12, no. 3 (2008): 51–72.

22. The humanists themselves referred to the program as the *studia humanitatis,* which consisted largely of the seven liberal arts, made up of the quadrivium (arithmetic, astronomy, geometry, and music) and the trivium (logic, rhetoric, and grammar).

23. See, e.g., Charles G. Nauert, *Humanism and the Culture of Renaissance Europe,* 2nd ed. (Cambridge, UK: Cambridge University Press, 2006); and William J. Bouwsma, "The Culture of Renaissance Humanism," *American Historical Association Pamphlet* (1973), 1–26.

Section I

The Lived Experience of Pain

1 The Current State of Pain in the United States

Two premises are needed to begin discussion on pain in American society: (1) pain is not adequately treated; and (2) pain ought to be adequately treated.[1] This chapter addresses the first premise above, which is an empirical claim.[2] The second premise asserts an ethical claim, which subsequent chapters will address.

THE PREVALENCE AND SCOPE OF PAIN IN AMERICAN SOCIETY

The statistics regarding pain in the U.S. are simply staggering. In the last eight years, two high-level national bodies charged with setting health priorities have issued lengthy reports on the prevalence and impact of pain in American society. First, in the summer of 2011 the Institute of Medicine ("IOM") released a report entitled *Relieving Pain in America*. In the report, the IOM notes that approximately 116 million U.S. adults experience chronic pain, a number that constitutes approximately one-third of the entire U.S. population.[3] Moreover, the IOM points out that this number is "a conservative estimate [of overall pain], as neither acute pain nor children are included" (2–6). Thus, chronic pain prevalence exceeds the prevalence of heart disease, diabetes, and cancer combined.

Presaging the 2011 IOM report, the National Center for Health Statistics (NCHS), focused on pain in its 2006 annual report on health in the U.S. The NCHS documented that over one-quarter of Americans (26 percent) aged 20 years and older reported a problem with pain of any kind that lasted more than 24 hours in the month prior to the interview (Figure 1.1).

As mentioned in the Introduction, the NCHS found that elderly persons were least likely to report pain (21 percent), which is especially troubling given the estimates of high pain prevalence among such populations.[4] The NCHS 2006 report notes that although elderly populations report pain less frequently than other classes of adults, "57 percent of older adults who reported pain indicated that the pain lasted for more than 1 year compared with 37 percent of adults 20–44 years of age who reported pain" (Figure 1.2).[5]

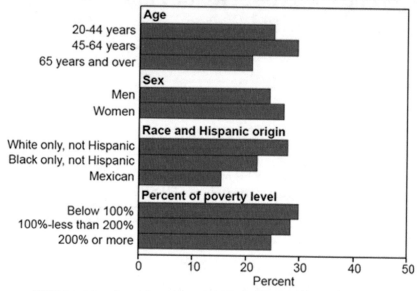

Figure 1.1   *Pain prevalence in the past month among adults 20 years old and older,*
1999–2002.

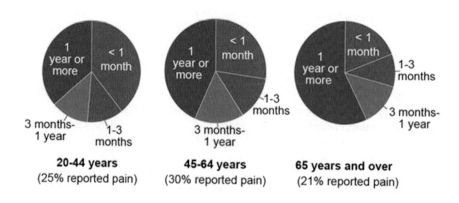

Figure 1.2   *Pain duration, 1999–2002.*

The 2006 NCHS Report breaks down pain prevalence by the type of pain. This breakdown is important because different kinds of pain seem to correlate with a better likelihood of receiving adequate treatment. For reasons that will be discussed in detail, there is good evidence that a person presenting, for example, with acute pain secondary to organic insult (such as from a car accident) stands a better chance of receiving adequate treatment for his/her pain than a person presenting in the same health care setting with chronic non-cancer pain.[6]

Pain is not monolithic. Different kinds of pain produce vastly different experiences for the pain sufferer in terms of, e.g., pain sensation (for example, burning, crushing, piercing), duration, prevalence, treatment, and stigma. Of the four types of pain (low back pain, migraine/severe headache, neck pain, and/or face pain) assessed in the 2006 NCHS Report, low back pain was the most prevalent overall and within each age group (Figure 1.3). This is significant because there is good evidence that low back pain is a particularly challenging chronic pain experience for providers, caregivers, and sufferers alike.[7] In addition, adults who reported low back pain lasting more than three months in 2004 reported worse health status than those who did not report such pain, regardless of age (Figure 1.4).

Migraine/severe headache occurred in 15 percent of the adults (Figure 1.4), but was particularly prevalent among women in their reproductive years, with roughly 25 percent of women aged 18–44 years reporting migraine/severe headache between 1997 and 2003.

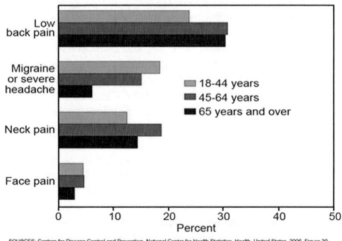

Low back, neck, migraine, face pain in past 3 months, 2004

SOURCES: Centers for Disease Control and Prevention, National Center for Health Statistics, Health, United States, 2006, Figure 30. Data from the National Health Interview Survey.

Figure 1.3   Low back, neck, migraine, and face pain in past 3 months, 2004.

Health status measures for adults with/without recent low back pain, 2004

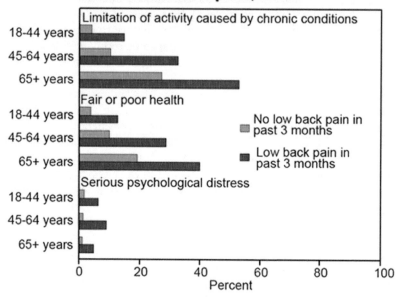

SOURCES: Centers for Disease Control and Prevention, National Center for Health Statistics, *Health, United States, 2006*, Figure 37. Data from the National Health Interview Survey.

Figure 1.4   Health status measures for adults with/without recent low back pain, 2004.

Thus, what the empirical evidence suggests about pain is not merely its prevalence, but how that prevalence varies across geographies of the individual body, in terms of differences in pain location, severity, and accompanying disability. Pain also varies across geographies of social groups, each of which has social worlds, histories, and practices of its own that are important in unpacking what pain experiences mean. Obviously relevant here is the explosive literature demonstrating inequities in and across multiple dimensions of health in the United States.[8] Pain is no exception to these general trends; not only do women suffer migraine/severe headache more frequently than men, but the NCHS Report found gender, age, and racial/ethnic differences in low back pain as well (Figure 1.3).

In addition, given the robust literature linking income and health,[9] it should be unsurprising that women of lower income levels were more likely to report pain (Figure 1.5). Pain inequalities began to attract significant attention in the early 1990s, prompting the Joint Commission to include pain guidelines in its accreditation requirements, and the Veterans Health Administration to introduce its own set of guidelines for the treatment of pain.[10] Yet, consistent with the trajectory of pain policy over the last 25 years, there is little indication that these efforts have alleviated inequalities in pain. The IOM cites dozens of studies documenting inequalities in diagnosing, assessing, and treating pain among various social and demographic categories including race, gender, income level, class, education, age (both children and the elderly), geographic location, veteran status, and cognitive status.[11] Moreover, like pain prevalence itself, pain inequalities are growing.

Specific reports of pain prevalence and treatment in certain populations particularly likely to experience pain (such as the elderly and veterans) paint an even more disturbing picture. A 2004 study reported that persistent non-malignant pain among nursing home residents in the U.S. was reliably estimated at a prevalence of 49–84 percent,[12] which is consistent with other studies.[13] As to veterans, there is a paucity of systematic data, and estimates of pain prevalence vary depending on the particular population under investigation, but several small studies report prevalence of 50 percent;[14] 47 percent;[15] and 78 percent (in a study of women veterans).[16]

The devastating inequalities in the treatment of pain are an urgent social and ethical issue. Thus, when I write of the need to ameliorate the under-treatment of pain, I refer not only to the efforts required to minimize the

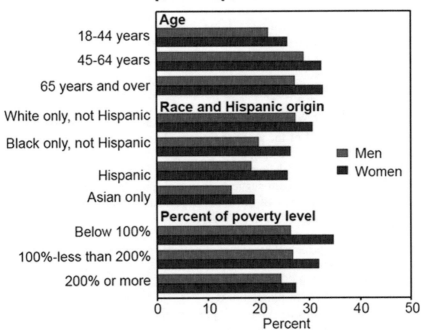

SOURCES: Centers for Disease Control and Prevention, National Center for Health Statistics, *Health, United States, 2006*, Figure 31. Data from the National Health Interview Survey.

Figure 1.5   Low back pain in last 3 months, 2004.

absolute burdens of pain in American society, but also to those needed to alleviate the inequitable distribution of pain. The need both to minimize pain and to compress pain inequalities reflects a particular approach to public health policies based on the work of British epidemiologist Sir Geoffrey Rose.[17] Rose's idea is that health policies should strive to maximize two goals: the improvement of overall population health, and the compression of health inequalities.[18] Health policies that advance both of these goals are generally preferable to policies that advance only one. As such, there are two goals for ethical, humane pain policy: to alleviate the absolute undertreatment of pain in the overall American population, and to compress the inequalities in the undertreatment of pain that disproportionately impacts marginalized and vulnerable subgroups.

Finally, the bulk of the data on pain prevalence addresses the reporting of pain, which is not equivalent to the experience of pain. This distinction exists at least in part because members of certain populations are significantly less likely to report pain even if they experience it. However, this fact actually strengthens the analysis, because the reasons why some communities might underreport their pain experiences are a key feature of the social and cultural discourses that shape and inform beliefs, attitudes, and practices towards such pain. To understand why elderly populations tend to underreport their pain requires some analysis of the meaning of pain in and among elderly populations.[19] My thesis here is that producing evidence-based pain policies that justify a hope that the undertreatment of pain can be ameliorated requires consideration of such social and cultural factors.

PREVALENCE VS. UNDERTREATMENT OF PAIN

Thus far, the evidence discussed in this chapter documents the high rates of pain prevalence and of inequalities in pain. There is little doubt that these rates imply failures in treating pain.

Chronic pain is by definition persistent or recurring. Therefore, high prevalence of chronic pain suggests that such pain is not being alleviated. Moreover, direct evidence of the undertreatment of pain is overwhelming. Resnik, Rehm, and Minard note that

> [p]ain is the principal reason why patients see physicians but it is routinely undertreated in health care. Many recent studies have demonstrated inadequate pain management in many different circumstances, including pain in terminal illness . . . pain in elderly populations . . . cancer pain . . . chronic pain . . . pain in emergency care . . . and postoperative pain . . .[20]

Also in 2001, Barry Furrow noted that "[p]ain is undertreated in the American health-care system at all levels: physician offices, hospitals, long-term care facilities."[21] C. Stratton Hill, Jr., a Texas-based pain physician who has devoted much of the last three decades to advocating locally, regionally, and nationally for improved treatment of pain, noted in 1995 that inadequate treatment for pain is the norm.[22] David Morris, whose work on pain is the chief inspiration for the approach employed in this book, observed in 1998 that "[f]or years, reliable studies have estimated the undertreatment for cancer pain at 50 percent of patients."[23] More recently, a 2009 study examined the adequacy of pain management practices between 1999 and 2006 in patients with bone metastases arising from terminal cancer, which are particularly painful. The authors concluded that, despite significant investment in and attention to cancer pain management, "there was no significant and perpetual decrease in the proportion of undermedicated patients over the seven-year study period. . . ."[24]

As I will discuss in Chapter 5 (this volume), there is reason to believe that pain resultant to visible lesions is likely to be treated better than pain that occurs in the absence of such perceptible pathologies (such as chronic pain). Given this, the fact that so many cancer patients suffer significant pain suggests that the undertreatment of chronic pain may be far worse. Precise data on the undertreatment of chronic pain is difficult to unearth. This is unsurprising given that chronic pain is generally contested, regardless of whose perspective is assessed (illness sufferer, provider, caregiver, policymaker, etc.).[25] Explaining why chronic pain is subject to such intense contest is a central objective of this book. But given that even the basic question of what qualifies as chronic pain promotes widespread disagreement, it is less surprising that there exist little data on the undertreatment of chronic pain. Nevertheless, Martino notes

> a widely shared and growing consensus in the medical and scientific communities . . . the law, social sciences, and humanities . . . and the popular press . . . that inadequate treatment of chronic pain is the rule in the United States and most developed nations.[26]

Any lingering doubts that pain is undertreated in the U.S. can be eliminated by review of the IOM Report on the undertreatment of pain, which noted simply that "[c]urrently, large numbers of Americans receive inadequate pain prevention, assessment, and treatment. . . ." (S-7). This fact formed the core charge for the IOM Committee tasked with researching and writing the Report, and drove the IOM to urge a "cultural transformation" regarding the treatment of pain.

Indeed, there is no serious suggestion that undertreatment of chronic pain is less of a problem than it once was. In 2009, Sean Morrison, one of the most recognizable palliative care physicians in the U.S., was queried regarding a number of studies documenting no improvement in pain management practices surveyed. Morrison expressed significant disappointment, stating that "[t]hese studies are particularly distressing as they indicate that so little progress has been made in the last decade in spite of substantial efforts to redress this situation."[27] Again, shedding some light on the social and cultural reasons for this lack of success is a central objective of this book.

Given these difficulties, there is little obvious reason to suspect dramatic advances in ameliorating the undertreatment of pain. One could respond to this doubt by noting that there exists a large and diverse community working to ameliorate the undertreatment of pain. However, such forces have converged on the issue for at least a quarter of a century, with little indication that the problems in treating pain in the U.S. have improved significantly.[28] Resnik, Rehm, and Minard observe that the undertreatment of pain

> is by no means a new problem in health care: for more than 25 years researchers have documented the undertreatment of pain. . . . In the last decade, many health care professionals (HCPs), professional organizations, and scholars have decried this problem and have championed the cause of better pain control.[29]

As mentioned in the Introduction, this well-intentioned social and cultural undertaking has involved diverse actors exchanging significant material, social, and technical resources, and has drawn the attention of some of the most wealthy and powerful organizations and institutions in the world (such as the U.S. government[30] and the multinational pharmaceutical industry[31]). Yet, for all these considerable inputs, the epidemiology of pain in the U.S. shows almost beyond question that these efforts have made little progress in improving one's chances of receiving adequate treatment for pain in the U.S.

Chapter 2 (this volume) begins the task of explaining how and why this is so.

NOTES

1. Goldberg, "The Sole Indexicality of Pain."
2. I do not provide here a complete epidemiologic account of pain in the U.S. Such an account would be lengthy and duplicative, since many of the sources and reports cited in this chapter already provide details.
3. IOM, *Relieving Pain in America,* 33.
4. Aida B. Won, Kate L. Lapane, Sue Vallow, Jeff Schein, John N. Morris, and Lewis A. Lipsitz, "Persistent Nonmalignant Pain and Analgesic Prescribing Patterns in Elderly Nursing Home Residents," *Journal of the American Geriatrics Society* 52, no. 6 (June 2004): 867–74; Joan M. Teno, Sherry Weitzen, Terrie Wetle, and Vincent Mor, "Persistent Pain in Nursing Home Residents," *Journal of the American Medical Association* 285, no. 16 (April 25, 2001): 2081; Bruce A. Ferrell, Betty R. Ferrell, and Lynne Rivera, "Pain in Cognitively Impaired Nursing Home Patients," *Journal of Pain and Symptom Management* 10, no. 8 (November 1995): 591–98.

5. National Center for Health Statistics, *Health United States 2006*, 70.
6. Jackson, "Stigma, Liminality, and Chronic Pain."
7. Lorna A. Rhodes, Carol A. McPhillips-Tangum, Christine Markham, and Rebecca Klenk, "The Power of the Visible: The Meaning of Diagnostic Tests in Chronic Back Pain," *Social Science & Medicine* 48, no. 9 (May 1999): 1189–203.
8. Staton, Panda, Chen, Genao, Kurz, Pasanen, Mechaber, Menon, O'Rorke, Wood, Rosenberg, Faeslis, Carey, Calleson, and Cykert, "When Race Matters"; Liana D. Castel, Benjamin R. Saville, Venita DePuy, Paul A. Godley, Katherine E. Hartmann, and Amy P. Abernethy, "Racial Differences in Pain During 1 Year among Women with Metastatic Breast Cancer," *Cancer* 112, no. 1 (January 1, 2008):162–70; Jeanette A. McNeill, Janice Reynolds, and Margaret L. Ney, "Unequal Quality of Cancer Pain Management: Disparity in Perceived Control and Proposed Solutions," *Oncology Nursing Forum* 34, no. 6 (November 2007): 1121–28; Mark J. Pletcher, Stefan G. Kertesz, Michael A. Kohn, and Ralph Gonzales, "Trends in Opioid Prescribing by Race/Ethnicity for Patients Seeking Care in US Emergency Departments," *Journal of the American Medical Association* 299, no. 1 (January 2, 2008): 70–8; Janet Kaye Heins, Alan Heins, Marianthe Grammas, Melissa Costello, Kun Huang, and Satya Mishra, "Disparities in Analgesia and Opioid Prescribing Practices for Patients with Musculoskeletal Pain in the Emergency Department," *Journal of Emergency Nursing* 32, no. 3 (June 2006): 219–24; Ian Chen, James Kurz, Mark Pasanen, Charles Faselis, Mukta Panda, Lisa J. Staton, Jane O'Rorke, Madhusudan Menon, Inginia Genao, JoAnn Wood, Alex J. Mechaber, Eric Rosenberg, Tim Carey, Diane Calleson, and Sam Cyker, "Racial Differences in Opioid Use for Chronic Nonmalignant Pain," *Journal of General Internal Medicine* 20, no. 7 (July 2005): 593–98; Louis D. Sullivan and Barry A. Eagel, "Leveling the Playing Field: Recognizing and Rectifying Disparities in Management of Pain," *Pain Medicine* 6, no. 1 (January 2005): 5–10; George Rust, Wendy N. Nembhard, Michelle Nichols, Folashade Omole, Patrick Minor, Gerrie Barosso, and Robert Mayberry, "Racial and Ethnic Disparities in the Provision of Epidural Analgesia to Georgia Medicaid Beneficiaries during Labor and Delivery," *American Journal of Obstetrics and Gynecology* 191, no. 2 (August 2004): 456–62; Carmen R. Green, Karen O. Anderson, Tamara A. Baker, Lisa C. Campbell, Sheila Decker, Roger B. Fillingim, Donna A. Kaloukalani, Kathryn E. Lasch, Cynthia Myers, Raymond C. Tait, Knox H. Todd, and April H. Vallerand, "The Unequal Burden of Pain: Confronting Racial and Ethnic Disparities in Pain," *Pain Medicine* 4, no. 3 (September 2003): 277–94; Vence L. Bonham, "Race, Ethnicity, and Pain Treatment: Striving to Understand the Causes and Solutions to the Disparities in Pain Treatment," *Journal of Law, Medicine & Ethics* 28, no. s4 (March 2001): 52–68.
9. See, e.g., Daniel S. Goldberg, "In Support of a Broad Model of Public Health: Disparities, Social Epidemiology and Public Health Causation," *Public Health Ethics* 2, no. 1 (April 2009): 70–83.
10. Kathryn Senior, "Racial Disparities in Pain Management in the USA," *Lancet Oncology* 9, no. 2 (February 2008): 96.
11. IOM, *Relieving Pain in America*.
12. Won, Lapane, Vallow, Schein, Morris, and Lipsitz, "Persistent Nonmalignant Pain and Analgesic Prescribing Patterns in Elderly Nursing Home Residents."
13. Ibid.; Teno, Weitzen, Wetle, and Mor, "Persistent Pain in Nursing Home Residents"; and Ferrell, Ferrell, and Rivera, "Pain in Cognitively Impaired Nursing Home Patients." The IOM estimated that 62 percent of nursing home residents experience persistent pain.

14. J. David Clark, "Chronic Pain Prevalence and Analgesic Prescribing in a General Medical Population," *Journal of Pain and Symptom Management* 23, no. 2 (February 2000): 131–37.
15. Ronald J. Gironda, Michael E. Clark, Jill P. Massengale, and Robyn L. Walker, "Pain among Veterans of Operations Enduring Freedom and Iraqi Freedom," *Pain Medicine* 7, no. 4 (July/August 2006): 339–43.
16. Sally G. Haskell, Alicia Heapy, M. Carrington Reid, Rebecca K. Papas, Robert D. Kerns, "The Prevalence and Age-Related Characteristics of Pain in a Sample of Women Veterans Receiving Primary Care," *Journal of Women's Health* 15, no. 7 (September 2006): 862–69.
17. Geoffrey Rose, *The Strategy of Preventive Medicine* (New York: Oxford University Press, 1992); Geoffrey Rose, "Sick Individuals and Sick Populations," *International Journal of Epidemiology* 14, no. 1 (1985): 32–8.
18. See, e.g., Joan Benach, Davide Malmusi, Yutaka Yasui, and José Miguel Martínez, "A New Typology of Policies to Tackle Health Inequalities and Scenarios of Impact Based On Rose's Population Approach," *Journal of Epidemiology & Community Health* 67, no. 3 (2013): 286–91.
19. Goldberg, "The Sole Indexicality of Pain."
20. Resnik, Rehm, and Minard, "The Undertreatment of Pain," 277 (citations omitted).
21. Barry R. Furrow, "Pain Management and Provider Liability: No More Excuses," *Journal of Law, Medicine & Ethics* 28, no. s4 (March 2001): 28.
22. C. Stratton Hill, Jr., "When Will Adequate Pain Management be the Norm?" *Journal of the American Medical Association* 274, no. 23 (December 20, 1995): 1881–82. This project benefits from the experience, counsel, and suggestions of Dr. Hill, to whom I am greatly indebted.
23. David B. Morris, *Illness and Culture in the Postmodern Age* (Berkeley, CA: University of California Press, 1998), 195.
24. Andrea M. Kirou-Mauro, Amanda Hird, Jennifer Wong, Emily Sinclair, Elizabeth A. Barnes, May Tsao, Cyril Danjoux, and Edward Chow, "Has Pain Management in Cancer Patients with Bone Metastases Improved? A Seven-Year Review at an Outpatient Palliative Radiotherapy Clinic," *Journal of Pain and Symptom Management* 37, no. 1 (January 2009): 82.
25. Jackson, "Stigma, Liminality, and Chronic Pain."
26. Ann M. Martino, "In Search of a New Ethic for Treating Patients with Chronic Pain: What Can Medical Boards Do?" *Journal of Law, Medicine & Ethics* 26, no. 4 (December 1998): 333 (citations omitted).
27. Sean Morrison, quoted in Senior, "Racial Disparities in Pain Management," 96.
28. Tousignant, "Pain and the Pursuit of Objectivity."
29. Resnik, Rehm, and Minard, "The Undertreatment of Pain," 276.
30. The NIH has showed particular interest in pain, establishing the NIH Pain Consortium in 1998, which is devoted to promoting collaboration in determining the optimal pain research agenda.
31. For example, Purdue Pharma and Endo Pharmaceuticals are two particularly visible and active supporters of improved pain management practices. The motivation for such support is another matter entirely, but the point is that significant private sector resources have been and continue to be marshaled in support of the treatment of pain.

2   The Lived Experience of Pain

INTRODUCTION

Pain is fundamental to our lived experiences as human beings. A painless existence is not conducive to human flourishing. Known as congenital analgesia, individuals who have this rare genetic disorder often suffer repeated injury, including broken bones, lacerated skin, damage to internal body tissues, and have significantly shortened life expectancy.[1] The point is that in whatever manifestation, pain is a fundamental part of human life. This is in part why a phenomenological approach to thinking about pain is so important. Such an approach expressly begins by refusing to abstract the phenomenon of pain from its context in the flow of lived experiences.

What is phenomenology? Although the word has a number of meanings, as applied to illness, the basic idea is that phenomenology is fundamentally a study of what the person exploring the illness feels and experiences in the flow of their own life. A phenomenology of illness addresses what it means for human beings, both individually and as part of social, familial, and communal networks, to live with an illness (and, if relevant, to die with one).

Improving the undertreatment of pain through policy is unlikely without a detailed understanding of the meaning of pain in American society. In large part, what has been sorely lacking from dominant approaches to the ethics and policy of pain is a thorough accounting of what pain means in the U.S. and why it takes on that particular constellation of meanings. A phenomenologic approach is crucial because it is expressly directed towards the goal of unpacking what the lived experience of pain is like for the sufferer, the caregiver, the provider, and other relevant stakeholders. Such an understanding forms the evidentiary basis for the policies offered in Chapter 8 (this volume).

PHENOMENOLOGY AND ILLNESS

First, a brief account of the phenomenology of illness itself is needed. Of course, there are experiences specific to any given illness that may not be generalizable to other types of illness experiences. For example, the phenomenology of ovarian cancer is qualitatively different from the phenomenology of type II diabetes. Nevertheless, there are, I submit, important insights into the experience of pain available in assessments of the general phenomenology of illness.

Eric Matthews's recent account of the problems in conceptualizing mental illness provides an excellent starting point in thinking through some aspects of the phenomenology of illness.[2] Matthews begins by explaining the materialist roots of the dominant medical model in conceptualizing psychiatric illness. For example, he notes that depression in psychiatry is frequently explained in terms of the accumulation of serotonin levels in the brain.[3] This frame is important to thinking about pain, because it tends to categorize a subjective phenomenon (here depression) in terms of a material, neurophysiological substrate. Similarly, in tracing the rise of the importance of diagnosis in psychiatry, Charles Rosenberg explains that

> [e]arlier interest in clinical description and postmortem pathology had articulated and disseminated a lesion-based theory of disease, but the late nineteenth century saw a hardening in this way of thinking, reflecting the assimilation of germ theories of infectious disease as well as a variety of findings from the laboratories of physiologists and biochemists.[4]

The key, as Rosenberg notes, is the "somatization" of mental illness during the nineteenth century, i.e., that "social legitimacy presumed somatic identity. . . ."[5] The importance of this modality in understanding the meaning of pain can hardly be overemphasized, and will be discussed in detail throughout this book. However, from a phenomenologic perspective, Matthews contends that, even if correct, the depression-serotonin explanation[6] fails to "help us understand any better why [the person] suffered from depression."[7] That is, even if we were certain that serotonin levels cause depression, we would still need "to understand the connection between these communication problems in the brain and the feelings of unworthiness intense enough to make one contemplate taking one's own life."[8]

In place of, or at least in addition to the tendencies of the dominant medical model to facilitate the reduction of illness experiences to material, "biological" entities and pathways, Matthews offers an account of illness that "relate[s] the meaning of concepts to its roots in the experience of subjects. What, after all, could, say, 'time' mean except what *we* meant by it?"[9] Such an account constitutes a phenomenology: "A phenomenological investigation of the meaning of concepts could not be separated from reflection on the consciousness which gave them meaning."[10] Moreover, a phenomenological approach eschews a focus on metaphysical questions, not because such inquiries are unimportant, but because they do not capture what it is like to actually experience the phenomenon. Matthews's point is to highlight the absurdity of the idea that the depression-serotonin causal explanation is literally equivalent to the subjective experience of depression. As Matthews puts it, the phenomenologist "seeks to *describe* our experience just as we have it. . . ."[11]

> In Heidegger's terms, we are unequivocally "beings-in-the-world." We should start, not from some ideal absolute, but from where we actually are. Our experience of the world is that of beings who are in the world, in some specific place and time, and for that very reason, experience or consciousness is not a matter of pure intellectual contemplation, but of active and emotional engagement with the world in various ways.[12]

Similarly, our lived experiences, the phenomena of our lives, are necessarily situated within social worlds and relationships; "[m]eanings are to be found, not by looking inside our own heads, but by investigating what we share with each other, in our common practical engagement with the world."[13] The phenomenologist rejects as absurd the idea that we can partition off our own subjectivity from our lived experiences of illness. Equally suspect is the related idea that from the perspective of knowledge production we *ought* to excise that subjectivity. This is what it means to "be in the world"; we are never outside of the world of our lived experiences. Matthews notes that "[s]ubjectivity, or mind, is not something detached from the world, but part of the world, interacting with objects rather than simply contemplating them."[14]

Thus in *Being and Time,* Heidegger observes that our "dealings" as beings-in-the-world are not "bare perceptual cognition, but rather that kind of concern which manipulates things and puts them to use; and this has its own kind of 'knowledge.'"[15] Heidegger emphasizes that as a discipline, biology is not concerned with the question of how the being-in-the-world makes meaning of its lived experiences,[16] but is rather, in Frederick Svenaeus's language, "focused on measuring the life-activities of objects in the world."[17] Heidegger observes the significant value in such practices, but argues that any attempt to understand how the subjects make meaning of their own lives and experiences in the world must proceed via entirely different pathways.[18] Similarly, Merleau-Ponty notes that "when I say that I see the house with my own eyes . . . I do not mean that my retina and crystalline lens, my eyes as material organs, go into action and cause me to see it; with only myself to consult, I can know nothing about this."[19] Merleau-Ponty's point is obviously not that the retina and material structures are irrelevant to vision, but rather that the experience of seeing is simply not reducible to such structures.[20]

The subjectivity central to the phenomenology of Heidegger and Merleau-Ponty is also crucial to thinking about illness and pain. It is impossible to assess the lived experience of illness and pain without accounting for the subjective understandings, feelings, and sensations that attend the illness or pain experience. The value of a phenomenological account of illness is precisely that the subjective experiences are the focus of the inquiry. A phenomenology of depression, for example, would tend to avoid detailed analyses of the biochemical and neurophysiological pathways of depression, because, however relevant those pathways might be to understanding the causation and treatment of depression, they have little to do with what it feels like to live with and experience depression.

So too does a phenomenology of pain attempt to account for the life-world of the pain sufferer. What is it like to suffer from pain? How is one's world constructed or taken apart in the face of pain? And because a phenomenological account understands 'being-in-the-world' in terms of our relationships with others, questions pertaining to the pain sufferer's social status and relationships with intimates, professional healers, and even perfect strangers take center stage.

THE PHENOMENOLOGY OF PAIN

So, what *is* it like to suffer from pain? There are numerous sources upon which to draw in answering this question, which is fortunate, for it signals that the value of a phenomenological approach to pain is recognized. Perhaps the seminal work is Elaine Scarry's *The Body in Pain*.[21] According to Scarry, pain silences. It destroys language and communication. It does this in large part because of what Scarry terms its "unsharability."[22] Pain is 'unsharable' because it is the quintessential private, subjective phenomenon. My pain is qualitatively distinct from your pain, even if our pain is caused by the same stimulus. As a corollary, there is an important sense in which others lack access to my pain. Scarry explains that "when one speaks about 'one's own physical pain' and about 'another person's physical pain,' one might appear to be talking about two wholly distinct orders of events."[23] She continues, "pain does not simply resist language, but actively destroys it, bringing about an immediate reversion to a state anterior to language, to the sounds and cries a human being makes before language is learned."[24]

While her perspective remains influential, many commentators reject Scarry's perspective on the private, unshareable nature of pain. For example, Mark Sullivan, exploring Wittgenstein's perspective, argues that pain itself is inherently social, and, as such, exists neither in minds or bodies but between them: "If pain acquires its meaning from use in dialogue, it may be most intelligible from the interpersonal point of view."[25] This explains why "[w]e are constantly socially negotiating as to what pain is or not."[26] Furthermore, Stan van Hooft notes that the mere fact that pain talk frequently involves figurative language does not imply its unshareability: "That one needs metaphors here does not imply that the experience is radically private, incommunicable, or unshareable."[27] Nevertheless, neither denies the silencing qualities of pain, which are generally well-recognized.[28]

As to those silencing qualities, communication and relationships between pain patients and their physicians are generally poor, with evidence of significant hostility between patients and providers.[29] Yet, given the social role of the physician as the savior[30] (also known as the rescue fantasy),[31] pain sufferers often maintain ambivalent feelings towards their physicians. Thomas and Johnson note that "the sufferer longs for a physician rescuer. Physicians are both trusted and mistrusted, with the pendulum swinging toward greater mistrust and alienation after repeated experiences of being unheard and unhealed."[32]

Pain does not just promote silence between patient and provider, but between pain sufferer and caregiver as well. In her ethnography of chronic pain patients, Jean Jackson notes that one of the patients remarked, "after a while, no one believes you. Even my wife."[33] The persistence of pain for weeks, months, and years may lead to caregiver exhaustion, a scenario in which the caregiver's capacity to hear and bear witness to the sufferer's pain erodes. Arthur Kleinman, Paul Brodwin, Byron Good, and Mary-Jo DelVecchio Good suggest that "[a]bsolute private certainty to the sufferer, pain may become absolute public doubt to the observer. The upshot is often a pervasive distrust that undermines family as well as clinical relationships."[34] Physician-anthropologist Marja-Liisa Honkasalo observes that "[s]everal of my informants say that social exclusion is the worst experience connected to chronic pain and that it is often felt as a punishment—they feel guilty for their condition and isolated from others."[35]

Yet, given the hope the suffering patient tends to invest in their physician, the alienation of the pain sufferer from their physician is in some sense even crueler than the silence that arises between the pain sufferer and his/her loved ones:

> Clearly, the most prominent others in narratives of pain patients, more significant than family members or friends, were physicians. Despite repeated experiences with doctors who were impersonal, unkind, or even cruel, participants [in the study] could not abandon a fantasy that there was a caring doctor out there somewhere who could provide relief for them.[36]

Pain also encourages silence because of typical reactions to pain behavior, which tend to stigmatize the pain sufferer. The pain sufferer's experiences with and fears of being stigmatized contributes to the silencing features of pain: "Participants generally kept the secret of having a chronically painful condition because they anticipated adverse outcomes if it were revealed. They perceived other people to have pejorative views of pain patients. They expected skepticism and disinterest rather than sympathy and support."[37]

Imposed silence is fundamentally isolating. Such alienation characterizes much of the lived experience of pain and of chronic pain in particular.[38] van

Hooft argues that what is unique about the phenomenology of pain is that it can isolate the pain sufferer in a "prison" of "their own suffering."[39]

Pain isolates because it paradoxically connects the sufferer to the body at the same time it separates the sufferer from the body. Outside of pain and illness experiences, our bodies are generally absent from our attention.[40] van Hooft observes that

> [i]nternal organs like the heart, lungs, or liver do their life-preserving work without calling attention to themselves in any way. Similarly, those parts of our body which we regularly use and can apprehend, such as our legs and hands, are absent from our attention as we use them. Our agency flows through them, as it were, and focuses upon the things in the world with which we are dealing.[41]

Drew Leder summarizes: "In our daily life we simply *are* our body, moving through the world as an integrated whole."[42] But pain disrupts this integration, often in sudden and terrible ways: "The body that was once silent now screams for attention. Where it once obeyed the least command, it now rebels against our desires and undermines our projects."[43]

The body in pain, then, becomes something grotesque and foreign: "For the painful body is already profoundly alien. Before coming to the doctor, the patient has already begun to objectify her body, poke and prod it, wonder at and resent its strange autonomy."[44] Leder notes the phenomenological paradox that pain presents: "Pain recalls us to our finitude and dependency, dragging us back into the mundane world. Yet this is a world in which we no longer feel at home."[45] Accordingly, pain isolates the sufferer not just from their providers and caregivers, but from themselves. "That to which we are most intimately connected becomes that from which we are most estranged."[46] Thomas and Johnson describe much of the dialogue in their study as "between the study participants and their nonhuman tormentor, the pain, more so than with other human beings. Participants described their pain as imprisoning them."[47]

Moreover, chronic pain patients often report a feeling of war or conflict with their own bodies. Milfrid Raheim and Wenche Haland characterize the experience of one chronic pain sufferer as "a feeling of being at the will of a treacherous body and left alone in never-ending pain. The body feels impossible to control."[48] This sufferer's "body is extremely objectified in her descriptions, experienced at a distance, pointing to an extreme disintegration between body and self, body and the practical world."[49] Svenaeus observes that "[i]n illness, the body is experienced as alien, as a 'broken tool' which gives rise to helplessness, resistance, and lack of control."[50] And Leder explains it thusly: "The mind thus experiences the Otherness of the physical."[51]

The phenomenologic account of (chronic) pain sketched here is, to say the least, not cheery.[52] The pain sufferer's lifeworld is often characterized by a variety of different kinds and sources of suffering. The pain sufferer may be isolated, often from his/her own body, may be silenced, may experience a profound rupture in their social and cultural worlds, and yet cannot escape the reality of their own pain experiences. Pain simultaneously exiles and separates the sufferer from their local worlds, but also swells to inhabit the geography of that world. Raheim and Haland describe how, for 'Maren,' "pain preoccupies her, disorganizing her world, leaving no place or time for relief. She describes an internal relation paradoxical in character, extreme distance toward her body and being totally absorbed by pain at the same time. Maren 'is pain' in radical meaning."[53] van Hooft notes that "pain crowds out all other interests and commitments. [Pain sufferers'] attention is focused upon themselves. . . . There is no reality for them but their own suffering. There is no subjectivity present to them but the nagging and searing insistence of their own tortured and isolated subjectivity."[54]

A phenomenology of pain is crucial because only by understanding the features of the pain sufferer's lifeworld can ethical strategies be developed for easing the existential suffering.[55] These strategies should themselves incorporate understanding of the crucial role of community in shaping lived experiences, including experiences of pain. Kleinman, Brodwin, Good, and Good argue that "[t]o regard pain as the experience of an individual, as it is regarded in standard biomedical practice, is so inadequate as to virtually assure inaccurate diagnosis and unsuccessful treatment."[56]

Indeed, exactly what the phenomenology of illness suggests is most absurd about dominant Western medical models—the attempt to carve out the role of subjectivity in the experience itself—is a prime characteristic of contemporary attitudes, beliefs, and practices towards pain, from providers, caregivers, and even pain sufferers themselves.

Accordingly, Isabelle Baszanger notes that

> [t]he development of anesthesia and the control of surgical pain it allowed, along with the emergence of effective therapeutic means, whether chemical or surgical . . . combined with the undeniable progress of anatomical, histological, and neurophysiological knowledge, reinforced the vision of pain as a signal or symptom that could reasonably be combated through the cause it indicated rather than for itself. In a sense, the approach to pain was confined to diagnosis and its difficult, more subjective aspects were excluded.[57]

It is the objects that cause pain, objects that facilitate diagnosis and causal attribution, that takes priority in most clinical encounters related to pain. Similarly, in his analysis of "pain talk" in the medical encounter, Christian Heath observes that

> [t]he cry of pain does not occasion sympathy or appreciation from the practitioner, nor is the actual experience of suffering by the patient

addressed as a topic in its own right. Rather the pain is managed within the framework of the diagnostic activity in which the doctor is engaged. The cry is treated as the basis for subsequent enquiries. . . . The practitioner maintains an analytic stance towards the suffering of the patient, a stance which arises from the necessity to make further enquiries in order to arrive at a diagnosis of the complaint.[58]

This is not to imply that the physician in this encounter is callous, but rather than the phenomenon of the patient's pain is important only insofar as it contributes to the reading of the signs, a reading which typically relies heavily on anatomical correlation.[59] Heath documents how the physician's body language and verbal cues permit the physician to "delicately sidestep . . . appreciation of the suffering and discourage . . . further cries of pain from the patient. In this way he is able to pursue the diagnostic enquiries at hand."[60] This observation resonates with Tolstoy's characterization of the physician in *The Death of Ivan Ilyich*:

To Ivan Ilyich, only one question mattered: was his condition serious or not? But the doctor ignored this inappropriate question. From his point of view it was an idle question and not worth considering. One simply had to weigh the alternatives: a floating kidney, chronic catarrh, or a disease of the caecum. It was not a matter of Ivan Ilyich's life but a conflict between a floating kidney and a disease of the caecum. And in Ivan Ilyich's presence the doctor resolved that conflict brilliantly in favor of the caecum.[61]

Similarly, Kleinman, Brodwin, Good, and Good observe that "[n]either in the biomedical research literature nor in the pain clinic does the *suffering* of pain patients and their intimate social circles receive much attention as such, that is, as a moral burden or a defining existential experience."[62]

Heath also explains that this dynamic does not implicate providers alone, but is a key device pain sufferers use in conceptualizing and understanding their pain. Thus, it is not simply that the physician alone sidesteps the sufferer's pain in the interests of making a diagnosis; the patient collaborates in this endeavor: "[T]he patient produces no further cries of pain. She withholds expression of her suffering and adopts an analytic or objective stance towards her own subjective experience . . . the patient is drawn into a particular framework of participation."[63] Honkasalo concurs, stating that the process of "diagnosis is morally crucial for the sufferers. . . . Patients are diligent pupils of learning biomedical language."[64] The importance of this point cannot be overemphasized, and will be a recurring theme throughout this book.

Furthermore, pain in the clinical encounter is understood by both providers and patients in terms of its location in a particular part of the body:

The actual expression of pain in the consultation . . . is in large part limited to certain relatively circumscribed diagnostic activities and in particular to occasions on [sic] which the practitioner is systematically attempting to identify the locale and thereby the nature of the patient's pain or suffering. Within the framework of these specific diagnostic activities, we can begin to discern the ways in which the revelation of pain is 'locally' organized.

In Honkasalo's research, "people spoke about body parts that were hurting and they searched for permanent localizations, names, and thus for moral relief from their situation."[66] Moreover, she observes, localization, or "attempt[s] to visualize and localize pain," is a feature of "medical diagnostics," and also "echoes patients' experiences."[67] The localizability of pain is a key aspect of the efforts to materialize pain, to carve out the lived experiences of pain, and hence the rise of localization in the nineteenth century is a vital part of the story I am trying to tell (and is a central subject of chapters 4 and 5, this volume).

Honkasalo observes that "clinicians often fail to take chronic pain seriously."[68] Her explanation for this finding is similar to Heath's emphasis on the significance of locating the pain in a particular anatomical space. Honkasalo notes that because communication about illness in the clinical encounter "is based on the visibility of causal connections and location . . . if [those parameters] fail, as in chronic pain, people's intensive experiences are not taken seriously."[69] Jackson notes that "the clinical perspective is the most authoritative discourse we have, so much so that other ways of talking about pain are automatically considered secondary or even suspect."[70] Even in context of providers, the attempt to downplay the subjective experience of pain is not limited to physicians; Carson and Mitchell observe that "[n]urses have been directed to try to manage pain as a problem instead of attending to the person who is living with the experience as the leader and teacher about how to live with pain when it is a persistent presence."[71]

Thus, if due attention to the phenomenology of pain is often missing in the clinical pain encounter, there exists for all stakeholders—including the pain sufferer him or herself—an opportunity to attend to the pain sufferer's lived experiences. This attention has ethical significance, as Carson and Mitchell suggest: "[U]nderstanding another's lived experience, especially the experience of a person in pain, is essential to any helping relationship."[72]

The key points here are (1) the importance of the attempt to understand what it is like to suffer pain; and (2) the unfortunate fact that these lived experiences of pain are not central in American biomedical encounters in which relief for pain is sought. Rather, as Heath documents, what takes priority in most of these encounters is the search for visible, material pathologies which are causing the sufferer's pain. Why? I neither claim nor believe that the pain sufferer's subjective experiences are minimized because providers are callous or uncaring. As demonstrated in this chapter, even the pain sufferers themselves participate in a dynamic that tends to minimize their own suffering and render its relevance a function of the search for visible, material pathologies.

Indeed, one of my central arguments is that an explanation of why the subjective experiences of pain are often missing or diminished in clinical encounters is vastly more complicated than a brute dichotomy between "good" and "bad" providers. Unpacking this complexity is the subject of Section II.

NOTES

1. Hirsch, Moye, and Dimon, "Congenital Indifference to Pain."
2. Eric Matthews, *Body-Subjects and Disordered Minds* (New York, NY: Oxford University Press, 2007).
3. Ibid., 60–9.
4. Charles E. Rosenberg, "Contested Boundaries: Psychiatry, Disease, and Diagnosis," *Perspectives in Biology and Medicine* 49, no. 6 (Summer 2006): 413.
5. Ibid., 414.
6. The endurance of the chemical imbalance theory of depression with little supporting evidence and significant contravening evidence makes for a fascinating example of the ways in which our notions of disease causality reveal much of social and cultural significance. I tend to agree with Arikha's suggestion that the persistence of this causal attribution may signal the continued influence of the humoral theory. Noga Arikha, *Passions & Tempers: A History of the Humours* (New York, NY: Harper Perennial, 2007).
7. Matthews, "Body-Subjects," 65.
8. Ibid. John Searle makes a similar argument in defending his account of consciousness, which I will address in Chapter 6 (this volume). Moreover, this is to say nothing of the omnipresence of the fallacy confusing correlation with causation in the chemical imbalance theory, about which Jeffrey R. Lacasse and Jonathan Leo have written extensively. Jeffrey R. Lacasse and Jonathan Leo, "The Media and the Chemical Imbalance Theory of Depression," *Society* 45, no. 1 (February 2008): 35–45; Jeffrey R. Lacasse and Jonathan Leo, "Serotonin and Depression: A Disconnect between the Advertisements and the Scientific Literature," *PLoS Medicine* 2, no. 12 (2005): e392, accessed June 5, 2009, from http://www.plosmedicine.org/article/info:doi/10.1371/journal.pmed.0020392; Jonathan Leo, "The Chemical Theory of Mental Illness," *Telos* 122 (Winter 2002): 169–77.
9. Matthews, "Body-Subjects," 81.
10. Ibid.
11. Ibid., 82.
12. Ibid., 85.
13. Ibid., 88.
14. Ibid.
15. Martin Heidegger, *Being and Time*, trans. John Macquarrie and Edward Robinson (San Francisco, CA: Harper Books, 1962), 95.
16. Heidegger, *Being and Time*, 75.
17. Frederick Svenaeus, "The Body Uncanny-Further Steps Towards a Phenomenology of Illness," *Medicine, Health Care and Philosophy* 3, no. 2 (May 2000): 127.
18. Heidegger, *Being and Time*, 71–5.

19. Maurice Merleau-Ponty, *Phenomenology of Perception,* trans. Colin Smith (London, UK: Routledge Press, 2002).

20. I will take up this argument again in earnest in Chapter 5 (this volume).

21. Elaine Scarry, *The Body In Pain: The Making and Unmaking of the World* (New York: Oxford University Press, 1985).

22. Ibid., 4.

23. Ibid.

24. Ibid.

25. Mark D Sullivan, "Finding Pain Between Minds and Bodies," *The Clinical Journal of Pain* 17, no. 2 (June 2001): 151. Though Wittgenstein's work is not the subject of this project, the philosophy, if it can be called such, of later Wittgenstein deeply influences all of my scholarship. The fact that Wittgenstein was fascinated with and expressly wrote on pain makes him even more relevant, and I hope to address his analysis in future work. The primary reason I have not addressed Wittgenstein in detail here is because of the complexity involved in any attempt to extricate Wittgenstein's specific perspective, and because any analysis that mentions Wittgenstein tends in due course to wholly become an analysis of Wittgenstein's perspective. I enthusiastically endorse the premise that his work virtually always deserves such attention, but that notion suggests this project would quickly transform into a Wittgensteinian account were I to address his writings on pain in any detail. In any case, Sullivan's 2001 essay is an excellent introduction to some of the implications of Wittgenstein's writings on pain.

26. Ibid.

27. Stan van Hooft, "Pain and Communication," *Medicine, Health Care and Philosophy* 6, no. 3 (October 2003): 257.

28. See Daniel S. Goldberg, "Exilic Effects of Illness and Pain in Solzhenitsyn's Cancer Ward: How Sharpening the Moral Imagination Can Facilitate Repatriation," *Journal of Medical Humanities* 30, no. 1 (March 2009): 29–42; Goldberg, "The Sole Indexicality of Pain."

29. Jackson, "Stigma, Liminality, and Chronic Pain"; Angela Byrne, Juliet Morton, and Peter Salmon, "Defending Against Patients' Pain: A Qualitative Analysis of Nurses' Responses to Children's Postoperative Pain," *Journal of Psychosomatic Research* 50, no. 2 (February 2001): 69–76.

30. See Goldberg, "Religion, the Culture of Biomedicine, and the Tremendum."

31. Howard Brody, *The Healer's Power* (New Haven, CT: Yale University Press), 137–56.

32. Thomas and Johnson, "A Phenomenologic Study of Chronic Pain."

33. Jackson, "After a While No One Believes You," 151.

34. Arthur Kleinman, Paul E. Brodwin, Byron J. Good, and Mary-Jo DelVecchio Good. "Pain as Human Experience: An Introduction," in *Pain as Human Experience,* eds. Paul E. Brodwin, Arthur Kleinman, Byron J. Good, and Mary-Jo DelVecchio Good (Berkeley, CA: University of California Press, 1992), 5.

35. Marja-Liisa Honkasalo, "What is Chronic is Ambiguity: Encountering Biomedicine with Long-Lasting Pain," *Journal of the Finnish Anthropological Society* 24, no. 4 (1999): 79.

36. Thomas and Johnson, "A Phenomenologic Study of Chronic Pain," 692.

37. Ibid., 691.

38. Daniel S. Goldberg, "Exilic Effects of Illness and Pain in Solzhenitsyn's Cancer Ward: How Sharpening the Moral Imagination Can Facilitate Repatriation," *Journal of Medical Humanities* 30, no. 1 (March 2009): 29–42; Drew Leder, "The Experience of Pain and Its Clinical Implications," in *The Ethics of Diagnosis,* eds. Jose Luis Peset and Diego Gracia (Dordrecht, Netherlands: Kluwer Academic Publishers, 1992), 95–106.

39. van Hooft, "Pain and Communication," 259.
40. Leder, *The Absent Body.*
41. van Hooft, "Pain and Communication," 256.
42. Leder, "The Experience of Pain," 98.
43. Ibid.
44. Ibid.
45. Ibid.
46. Ibid.
47. Thomas and Johnson, "A Phenomenologic Study of Chronic Pain," 692.
48. Milfrid Raheim and Wenche Haland, "Lived Experience of Chronic Pain and Fibromyalgia: Women's Stories from Daily Life," *Qualitative Health Research* 16, no. 6 (July 2006): 748.
49. Ibid., 753.
50. Svenaeus, "The Body Uncanny," 134.
51. Leder, "The Experience of Pain," 92.
52. For reasons discussed in the Preface, I am less interested in the redemptive possibilities of pain, though I do not deny the existence or the power of such a meaning-making device.
53. Raheim and Haland, "Lived Experience of Chronic Pain," 753.
54. van Hooft, "Pain and Communication," 259.
55. I will detail these strategies in Chapter 7 (this volume), in which I discuss my recommendations for ethical, evidence-based pain policy.
56. Kleinman, Brodwin, Good, and Good, "Pain as Human Experience: An Introduction," 9.
57. Bazsanger, *Inventing Pain Medicine,* 29.
58. Christian Heath, "Pain Talk: The Expression of Suffering in the Medical Consultation," *Social Psychology Quarterly* 52, no. 2 (June 1989): 115–16.
59. The role of anatomy in shaping the meaning of pain is paramount, and will be addressed in detail in chapters 3 and 4 (this volume).
60. Heath, 116.
61. Leo Tolstoy, *The Death of Ivan Ilyich,* trans. Lynn Soloaroff (New York: Bantam Books, 1981), 65.
62. Kleinman, Brodwin, Good, and Good, "Pain as Human Experience," 14 (emphasis in original).
63. Heath, "Pain Talk," 116.
64. Marja-Liisa Honkasalo, "Chronic Pain as a Posture Towards the World," *Scandinavian Journal of Psychology* 41, no. 3 (September 2000): 204.
65. Heath, "Pain Talk," 122.
66. Honkasalo, "Chronic Pain as a Posture," 204.
67. Honkasalo, "What is Chronic is Ambiguity," 80.
68. Honkasalo, "Chronic Pain as a Posture," 198.
69. Honkasalo, "What is Chronic is Ambiguity," 40.
70. Jackson, "Stigma, Liminality, and Chronic Pain," 15.
71. M. Gail Carson and Gail J. Mitchell, "The Experience of Living with Persistent Pain," *Journal of Advanced Nursing* 28, no. 6 (December 1998): 1243.
72. Ibid.

Section II

History, the Power of the Visible, and Pain

3 The History of Pain without Lesion in Mid- to Late-Nineteenth-Century America

INTRODUCTION

History matters. And history does not matter solely in order to understand events, ideas, and conditions in their own historical context. History is also critical for understanding contemporary affairs. The argument of this book is that trying to ameliorate the undertreatment of pain is unlikely without a deep understanding of what pain means in American society. This section develops a supporting claim: attempting to understand the meanings of pain without thinking about the history of pain is like studying a leaf without awareness of the tree to which it belongs. As Hill suggests, beliefs and attitudes about pain have been "systematically transferred from one generation of physicians to another."[1]

Hence this chapter begins the task of explaining the critical importance of the history of pain in American society by examining one particular phenomenon in the mid- to late nineteenth century: attitudes, practices, and beliefs of pioneering American neurologists towards patients' experiences of pain without lesion. The following chapter substantiates the crucial historical link between then and now, and explains why these nineteenth-century attitudes, practices, and beliefs are so important both for understanding the contemporary undertreatment of pain in American society, and for offering ethical policy prescriptions.

My primary thesis is that pain is treated so poorly in American society because it typically does not present with discrete material pathologies—i.e., lesions in the brain and nervous system—that can be clinically correlated with the experience of pain. Supporting this claim requires historical analysis of how and why seeing such pathologies came to be so important within both American biomedical culture and even within American culture in general. What follows here, however, is not a detailed contribution to the history of medicine regarding neurology and pain without lesion. The express historical argument that makes extensive use of available primary sources is available elsewhere.[2] Instead, chapters 3 and 4 (this volume) constitute an attempt to synthesize some of the key intellectual history of medicine in the nineteenth-century U.S. that bears specifically on matters of pain, mind, body, and brain, and to show its continued relevance to the present.

PAIN WITHOUT LESION: DEBATE AMONG AMERICAN NEUROLOGISTS, 1850–1900

In his 1887 treatise on spinal irritation, American neurologist William A. Hammond observed that he would endeavor 'not to claim too much for a pathological condition which I am very sure exists, and which I therefore think is entitled to recognition.'[3] The fact that Hammond, who was unquestionably one of the most important physicians in the U.S. during the latter half of the nineteenth century, begins his exposition by assuring readers that spinal irritation does in fact exist implies his awareness that some members of his intended audience might harbor doubts. Moreover, Hammond's choice of language is critical; he does not assert a nosological claim that the *disease* of spinal irritation exists, but rather advances a morphological/ anatomical claim, that the 'pathological condition exists.' The linking of the disease entity to its pathological condition suggests that the nosological reality is a function of its pathological anatomy. Where a discrete, material lesion exists that can be clinically correlated with a patient's illness complaint, the disease exists and is entitled to recognition.

The central claim is that leading neurologists of the time generally denied the possibility that pain could exist in the absence of material lesion. However, there is little support for the idea that American physicians of the time ignored or trivialized the pain experiences of their patients. Indeed, given the Victorian emphasis on suffering and sympathy, such behavior would have been especially taboo, at least with regards to socially privileged patients. On the other hand, the fact that American neurologists were aware of and sensitive to their patients' pain does not imply that they allowed that such pain could exist in the absence of a material (morbid) lesion. I contend that American neurologists followed their European counterparts in repeatedly insisting that if the patient experiences pain, then such a lesion must perforce exist, even if medical techniques of the time simply did not permit discernment of the lesion itself.

There are at least two reasons for focusing on neurologists. First, because many of the different experiences of pain without lesion implicated concerns related to the brain and the nervous system, early neurologists often treated nineteenth-century pain sufferers. As the neurologists themselves asserted, the 'seat of disease' for many kinds of pain without lesion was located in the nervous system, and hence was properly deemed within their purview. Second, and related, because so many experiences of pain without lesion implicated the brain and the nervous system, attitudes, practices, and beliefs among early neurologists regarding the mind-body relationship are important areas for investigation.[4] Chapter 5 (this volume) expressly takes up analysis of the role mind-body dualism plays in shaping the contemporary undertreatment of pain, thereby connecting past and present attitudes, practices, and beliefs regarding pain.

It is well-known that pain is far and away the most common complaint contemporary American patients bring to their physicians; there is little reason to believe that pain was significantly less common an experience for people living in the nineteenth century. The argument, therefore, is that understanding something about the attitudes and beliefs of the physicians treating them merits study. Understanding these attitudes and beliefs in turn requires a basic understanding of the sea changes in Western allopathic medicine that occurred during the nineteenth century.

PATHOLOGICAL ANATOMY AND
THE BIRTH OF THE CLINIC

In *The Birth of the Clinic,* Michel Foucault argues that, at the turn of the nineteenth century, in one of the centers of Western medicine (Paris), a group of scientists and physicians began to formulate a model of health and disease that would come to be called the anatomoclinical method.[5] Foucault's answer to the implicit question in the title of his book (how was the clinic born?) is premised on an understanding of the ideas, conceptions, and conditions that preceded it. To understand the nineteenth-century changes in medical practice, disease, health, and ultimately, in pain, it is necessary to think about earlier conceptions of disease and the body.

Nicholas D. Jewson notes that 'bedside medicine' in the late eighteenth century 'was polycentric and polymorphous . . . medical knowledge consisted of a chaotic diversity of schools of thought. The definition of the field was diffuse and problematic, disciplinary boundaries weak and amorphous.'[6] Even allowing for such complexity, however, it is not impossible to discern some important themes and patterns among competing medical cosmologies.[7]

In contrast to the emphasis on discrete material lesions featuring prominently in the Paris School of the nineteenth century, earlier healers working in the humoral tradition tended to eschew the importance of material localization in thinking about illness. The 'morbid forces [that caused disease] were located within the context of the total body system rather than any particular organ or tissue.'[8] Prior to the nineteenth century, prevailing medical cosmologies promoted a holistic conception, one predicated on humoral balance rather than on local pathologies. Physician and historian Robert Martensen notes that '[i]n a humoral schema, none of the solid tissues of the body were as important as the body's hollow spaces. These spaces contained the humors and humors had physiologic agency.'[9]

The emphasis on the illness sufferer's lifeworld, on a holistic notion of the interplay between subject and illness, is also evident in humoral understandings of pain. Lisa Wynne Smith's analysis of several sets of eighteenth-century medical consultations confirms the general medical cosmologies attributed here to a humoral schema. The language of pain in these letters 'was extraordinarily descriptive and personal. Humoralism fundamentally shaped sufferers' experience of their bodies, as revealed by descriptions of internal sensations and mind/body overlap.'[10] Specifically,

> [s]uffering had a flexible vocabulary, concurrently describing physical and emotional pains in ways that underscore the anxiety surrounding illness. This emphasizes the extent to which body and mind were inseparable in the early eighteenth century; pain involved one's whole being, both body and soul. Patients and their doctors often referred to emotional states as symptoms.[11]

Thus one early modern physician linked his clinical diagnosis 'with the patient's perceptions, which appear plainly–"sinking at the heart." While it was a physical problem, the term also indicated an emotion when alongside symptoms like 'heavy disposition' and 'dejection of spirit."[12]

This early modern linkage of body and soul in context of pain has older roots. Esther Cohen observes that '[a]ll major late medieval discourses on pain—in theology, medicine, and law—viewed "physical" pain as a function of the soul.'[13] Erected primarily on Augustinian foundations, pain was inextricably linked with guilt and fear.[14] Augustine explained the martyrs' lack of pain on this basis; they, like the Virgin Mary herself, did not suffer pain because they were free of guilt and fear.[15] 'The message was clear: pain lay in the soul; it resulted from the soul's sin and guilt, and its awareness of that guilt, of the ensuing retribution, and of the fear thereof.'[16]

The key point in the humoral conception of pain was the fundamental enmeshment of 'physical' and 'emotional' pain, of mind, body, and soul.[17] Consistent with humoral medical cosmologies, the subjectivity of the patient's lived experiences were inseparable from illness and pain. However, this is not to suggest that the concept of pain in humoral schemes was unproblematic. The connection between expressions of pain and truth challenged persons and communities from the Middle Ages to the early modern period, and the best evidence of this is in the practice of torture.[18] Cohen observes that 'for the physician, expressions of pain led to the truth of illness, and for the theologian, to the truth of sin and salvation.' 'Torture was thought to work because of the close relationship between body and soul; the truth of the soul could be forced out through physical pain.'[19] Writing about the relationship between pain, torture, and truth in early modern France, Lisa Silverman explains that

> [t]ruth is lodged in the matter of the body; judges were required to draw it out (tirer) or extract it (arracher) from the body, just as tears and teeth

are drawn. Truth resides in the flesh itself and must be torn out of that flesh piece by piece. . . . Pain is . . . the vehicle of truth-telling, a distillation of the pure substance lodged in the impure flesh.[20]

However, while the interplay between pain, suffering, guilt, and truth are complex and challenging, there is in humoralism a unity between 'physical' pain and mental or emotional experiences such as suffering, guilt, and fear. In comparison, the importance of pathological anatomy to the practice of medicine during the nineteenth century signals a sea change. Disease began to be conceptualized in a different sense, and a novel medical cosmology predicated on local, discrete entities as the cause of disease began to be not simply studied, but *practiced*.[21]

Foucault observes that

> [a]t a very early stage historians linked the new medical spirit with the discovery of pathological anatomy, which seemed to define it in its essentials, to bear it and overlap it, to form both its most vital expression and its deepest reason.[22]

While there is general acceptance among historians that anatomy gradually became more important during the early modern era, it was not until the nineteenth century that it would begin to take on a central role in defining medical practice.[23] Foucault even terms the new method the 'anatomo-clinical' method, and his locution remains the norm.

Foucault characterizes this change:

> The appearance of the clinic as a historical fact must be identified with the system of these reorganizations. This new structure is indicated— but not, of course, exhausted—by the minute but decisive change, whereby the question: 'What is the matter with you?', with which the eighteenth-century dialogue between doctor and patient began (a dialogue possessing its own grammar and style), was replaced by that other question: 'Where does it hurt?', in which we recognize the operation of the clinic and the principle of its entire discourse.'[24]

Foucault's point is that the birth of the clinic is linked the capacity to localize discrete agents of disease to specific places, structures, and tissues inside the body. Whereas prior to the nineteenth century, tissues were far less important than the hollow channels through which humors flowed,[25] this conceptual geography was inverted during the nineteenth century. This inversion shows the importance of pathological anatomy to the birth of clinical method. Indeed, Martensen goes so far as to suggest that 'Western learned medicine's most distinctive knowledge-making feature has been its historic reliance on anatomy.'[26] In a particularly revealing passage, Elizabeth

Hurren notes the changing conceptions of cadavers in the Oxford anatomy department of the late nineteenth century:

> When the department opened, every body taken for dissection was named, and funeral expenses were recorded individually. After ten years, during which the department expanded, the bodies were no longer named but instead were numbered. Finally, once the department was fully established, each pauper was simply recorded as 'material' or 'subject.'[27]

Hurren concludes that '[a]t each stage in the development of Oxford's cadaver business, reductionist language evolved. In a literal sense, the poor had become objects of material interest, rather than individual cases.'[28]

But the importance of Foucault's analysis extends well beyond a simple explanation of the role of anatomy in shaping modern clinical method. Foucault is interested in medical perception. Anatomy was so important to the birth of the clinic because of what the investigating, clinical Eye could *see* through such practice. As such, a crucial rhetorical device Foucault uses to explain the birth of the clinic is what he refers to as the 'clinical gaze' that connects lesions and illness complaints. Foucault's conception is not meant to be taken literally; the importance of physically seeing the signs of illness was understood long before the nineteenth century.[29] But the clinical gaze itself did mark something fundamentally distinct from the medical cosmologies that preceded it. As historian Roselyne Ray observes in context of pain,

> [a]t the dawn of the nineteenth century, physicians were looking for a pure sign which would remove the ambiguities inherent in symptoms. They wished to find a sign, the meaning of which would be as certain as that provided by the lesion found at dissection.[30]

Moreover, nineteenth-century changes in medical culture had dramatic effects on the way pain was conceptualized.

THE INVISIBILITY OF PAIN

Literature scholar David Morris picks up the Foucauldian interpretation of the birth of the clinic in a 1998 essay that connects these nineteenth-century changes to pain in context of

> [a] revolutionary readjustment in the realms of the visible and the invisible. In effect, while a new clinically based scientific medical perception begins to make pain increasingly visible inside the body, pain outside the nervous system and outside the clinic begins to seem correspondingly invisible.[31]

His point is that the focus on tissue pathologies and structural lesions that shaped the anatomoclinical method meant that pain that was not visible inside the body began to vanish from sight. Morris further argues that

> Pain . . . becomes newly visible and objectified. The physician does not see the pain directly, of course, but the clinical gaze penetrates deep within the body to expose pain's hidden sources and processes. The lesion—illuminated, mapped, and verified—increasingly comes to represent pain as it is made newly visible to the gaze of the physician. As a corollary, what the gaze of the clinic cannot see, cannot verify, and cannot transform into an objectified visible image of pain becomes, so to speak, invisible.[32]

These are provocative claims, made without extensive analysis of primary sources. They have provoked fairly strong reactions among several pain scholars. Noémi Tousignant charges that Morris has 'caricatured the modern medically-dominated view of pain,' 'exaggerated the medicalisation of pain,' 'overestimated the power exercised by the medical establishment over the definition and the management of pain,' and 'oversimplified the medical view of pain.'[33] Psychiatrist Andrew Hodgkiss devotes an entire monograph to the repudiation of Morris's claims regarding visible and invisible pain.[34] Although in large part I accept these criticisms, the perspectives of Morris and his critics can in fact be reconciled. Nineteenth-century American neurologists did not trivialize or invalidate their (socially privileged) patients' pain; nevertheless, the idea that pain could exist in the absence of a discrete, material lesion becomes increasingly untenable over the course of the long nineteenth century.

The first step to understanding how this reconciliation is possible is assessing the impact of the specificity theory as to pain, a theory that was connected to developments in experimental physiology and electricity. Many nineteenth-century physicians and scientists discussed the potential and capacity of electricity to treat various kinds of pain.[35] Johannes Müller's discovery of the specialization of nerve fibers and the electrochemical conduction of signals is crucial because it facilitated the development of the specificity theory with regard to pain.[36]

The specificity theory is not one account, but is rather a general framework for the physiology of the nervous system. In its most basic form, the idea is that specific nerve fibers respond to specific stimuli and convey particular sensations related to the stimulus. This means that the application of cold, heat, and pain result in the activation of certain nerve fibers, but not others.[37] In addition to research on the sensory specificity of nerve fibers, French physiologists François Magendie and Claude Bernard emphasized the distinction between the specific control of the motor function of the spinal nerves' anterior roots and that of the sensory function of its posterior roots.[38]

The single most important facet of the specificity theory as to pain is the implication that it was generally localizable. Thus in describing neuralgia, which American neurologist James Leonard Corning defined as pain due to 'extra-cranial causes,' he notes the appearance of 'painful spots' which are 'present in the majority of cases of neuralgia,' and about which 'careful digital exploration will rarely fail to result in their accurate localization.'[39]

In late nineteenth-century discussions on neurology and pain, the concept of localization generally does not refer to the notion that an impression or sensation is caused by a nerve that exists proximal to the area in which the sensation is experienced. Rather, what is usually meant by 'localization' is the idea, quite foreign to humoral theory, that the material pathology causing the sensation is *localizable* to a discrete, specific point or area within the inner body.

Historian Noga Arikha uses the term 'locationism' to describe their attempts to correlate discrete material pathology with an observed sign.[40] This term further supports the idea that the term 'localization' in late nineteenth-century neurological texts on pain refers not to the proximity of the material pathology, but to the fact that such a pathology exists at a discrete location inside the body. Similarly, the fact that physicians of the time were well aware that gross cerebral lesions were capable of producing certain kinds of pain[41] is consistent with this concept of localization. This is because the attribution of pain to cerebral lesions links the symptom itself to a specific tissue pathology.

This is why Foucault's characterization of clinical medicine centers on medical perception: What did the clinical Eye perceive? What did it project as causing illness? Furthermore, causal attributions of disease are a significant window into social, cultural, and political beliefs.[42] That nineteenth-century physicians seemed to attribute many kinds of pain to disturbances in relevant tissues, whether 'irritation' of the nerves as in spinal irritation and neuralgia,[43] or to cerebral lesions, as in some forms of headache,[44] is important for what it indicates regarding the meaning of pain.

Given the significance of pathological anatomy to nineteenth-century medical thought, it is unsurprising that nineteenth-century neurologists found pain caused by gross lesions easy to diagnose (though not necessarily easy to treat).[45] This is at least in part because gross cerebral lesions tended to produce a number of other symptoms that contributed to the differential diagnosis, including 'progressive loss of muscular power, vertigo, visual impairment and derangement of the faculty of recollection.'[46] But what of pain that tended to occur in the absence of discoverable lesions? Corning observes in two of his texts that '[o]rganic disease is by no means as frequent a cause of headache as might be imagined from the percentage of gross cerebral lesions.'[47] How did leading neurologists conceive of pain without lesion during this period?

If one understands the term 'lesion' as more than the gross cerebral lesions that physicians had long known of, then the best answer is that leading neurologists did not conceive of it at all. This is certainly not to suggest that nineteenth-century American physicians were ignorant of pain without lesion, nor that they trivialized it.[48] Indeed, there is little support in virtually any primary sources for the proposition that physicians typically invalidated their patients' pain.

However, this observation must be qualified: it is socially privileged patients whose pain was more likely to be legitimized and acknowledged. Like most forms of medical care, nineteenth-century regard and treatment for pain was distributed according to a number of different social strata, including class, race, age, gender, occupation, and other indicia of social status and hierarchy. Thus, for example, Martin Pernick pointed out over a generation ago that a complex moral calculus governed the dispensation of analgesia in nineteenth-century America, and predictably, members of marginalized groups in American society (e.g., African-Americans, the poor) were less likely to be administered analgesia.[49] Many of these patterns are rather obviously connected to individual and institutional racism, which, as Keith Wailoo has shown, had profound effects for the treatment of African-Americans' pain into the twentieth century as well.[50]

Furthermore, while it is generally correct to note that socially privileged patients' pain was not ignored by nineteenth-century physicians in either Europe or in the U.S., there are well-documented exceptions, such as the case of railway spine or spinal concussion. In both Great Britain and the U.S., many physicians and neurologists rejected injured workers and railway passengers' complaints of injury following railway accidents.[51]

But even with these qualifications, the general proposition that nineteenth-century neurologists did not ignore or trivialize their socially privileged patients' pain is generally correct. However, the claim Morris advances is that pain without lesion becomes invisible during the nineteenth century. A number of leading nineteenth-century physicians and neurologists suggested that even pain that seemed to appear in the absence of any lesions must nevertheless feature such lesions. As an object of inquiry, then, pain without pathology in some kind of tissue ceases to exist in the clinical gaze.

One of the best sources for locating this view is Hammond's treatise on spinal irritation. Hammond is one of the progenitors of American neurology and a founder of the American Neurology Association.[52] His views on pain without lesion are therefore particularly important. Nineteenth-century physicians were quite aware of the existence of pain that seemed to persist in the absence of any identifiable lesion. Accordingly, Hammond has no patience for those who reject the disease known as 'spinal irritation,' suggesting that those who do so must have limited experience "and therefore they cannot see; or they must have been endowed either with restricted powers of observation or with minds so constituted as to cause them wilfully to close their eyes to the facts that they did not care to see."[53]

In referring to those who 'cannot see,' who have 'restricted powers of observation,' and who 'close their eyes to the facts that they did not care to see,' Hammond emphasizes the power of clinical sight in validating spinal irritation.[54] Yet, the fact that Hammond undoubtedly believed in the existence of spinal irritation does not imply that he countenanced the existence of pain without any material pathology. In spite of his acknowledgment that anatomical work revealed no gross lesions or pathologies that would account for the pain of spinal irritation, Hammond did not hesitate to localize the causes of such pain to lesions in various regions of the spinal cord.[55]

This excerpt also demonstrates the work that the concept of localization performs in Hammond's medical cosmology; the issue is not whether the material pathology exists, but is simply where the lesion can be localized. In the case of spinal irritation, Hammond concedes that no obvious spinal lesions can be found at postmortem.[56] However, not just in this case, but in 'all cases' in which correlation of disease and pathological anatomy is unavailing, Hammond insists that it is appropriate to construct a hypothesis of the 'real nature' of the disease.[57] There is little doubt that the 'real nature' of spinal irritation is a reference to the specific lesion to which he attributes causation. In fact, Hammond notes that the general failure to locate the lesion that causes spinal irritation at post-mortem does not imply its nonexistence. On the contrary, given the localization of lesions, it is likely that the seat of disease exists at some specific region in the spinal cord or central nervous system.[58]

Thus, Hammond's argument is that the seat of spinal irritation is localizable in a lesion that exists somewhere in the spinal cord, but whose precise location and character has not yet been ascertained.[59]

The power of the lesion in the construction of pain is such that the possibility that pain might exist without a lesion is not tenable for Hammond. This does not mean that Hammond denies the existence of spinal irritation; it does mean that he denies the existence of a disease entity named 'spinal irritation' without a concomitant tissue pathology of some sort. Accordingly, there is for him no such clinical entity as pain from spinal irritation that cannot be located in a tissue pathology.

As historian Bonnie Ellen Blustein points out, however, Hammond was a particularly committed reductionist as to the role material structure played in defining illness.[60] Thus, if Hammond's views on pain without lesion are isolated, that may diminish the strength of the claim regarding the power of the visible lesion in late nineteenth-century American neurological discourse on pain. As it turns out, Hammond's views were typical. His account of pain without lesion—that it in fact is pain *with* (undiscovered) lesion—appears throughout nineteenth-century American texts on pain.[61] Moreover, like Hammond, nineteenth-century neurologists emphasized that pathological anatomical changes correlated with pain were simply not visible either to the naked eye or via microscope.[62] This emphasis on the technical gaps preventing *visibility* of the lesions presages the importance of the subsequent use of medical imaging techniques in illuminating features of the inner body that were previously undiscoverable—X-rays, electroencephalography, tomographic techniques, and, of late, fMRI.

What these sources demonstrate regarding the notion of pain without lesion is its incoherence. Severe chronic pain most certainly 'existed' in the eyes of these healers, and the general humanitarian impulse of the nineteenth century prompted widespread social and cultural concern with pain and suffering itself.[63] The key point is neither that pain without lesion was ignored or trivialized nor that American physicians failed to appreciate the depth of their patients' suffering. Rather, the crucial point is the link between material tissue pathology and pain. That chronic, intractable, difficult pain could exist without lesion as a primary causal factor was untenable, so much so that leading American neurologists were prepared simply to assume the existence of a lesion in a specific location in the body. Pain itself becomes a material problem, in the sense that its existence seemed to be predicated on the existence of a localized tissue pathology that causes the pain.

CONCLUSION

The analysis developed in this chapter lies at the core of the book. My argument is that the extensive efforts to improve the treatment of pain have generally had little effect because such efforts have not been linked to an understanding of the meaning of pain in American society. In turn, no such understanding of the meaning of pain is possible without thinking about how historical attitudes, practices, and beliefs towards pain that generally resists the "ocular demonstrations"[64] that animate modern clinical method, shape and inform the multiple meanings of pain in American society. Having illustrated how the emphasis on visible pathologies in material structures and tissues within the body were key to conceptualizing pain without lesion among leading late nineteenth-century American neurologists, Chapter 4 (this volume) moves on to explain how this history manifests in contemporary clinical medicine in the U.S.

NOTES

1. Hill, "When Will Adequate Pain Management be the Norm," 1881.
2. Daniel S. Goldberg, "Pain Without Lesion: Debate Among American Neurologists, 1850–1900," *19: Interdisciplinary Studies in the Long Nineteenth Century* 15 (2012), available at http://19.bbk.ac.uk/index.php/19/article/view/629.
3. William A. Hammond, *Spinal Irritation* (Detroit, MI: George S. Davis, 1886), 19.
4. Time and space preclude discussion of mind-body dualism in late nineteenth-century American neurology in this essay. I mention it here as a way of justifying the focus on neurologists.
5. There exists controversy over the extent to which the changes at issue here occurred uniquely in Paris, or whether antecedent and similar contemporary developments occurred in England of the time. See, e.g., Othmar Keel, "Was Anatomical and Tissue Pathology a Product of the Paris Clinical School or Not?" in *Constructing Paris Medicine*, eds. Caroline Hannaway and Ann F.

LaBerge (Amsterdam: Rodopi Press, 1998), 117–84. This debate is not material to my analysis because the subject of my inquiry is the ideas that arise out of the Paris School. Insofar as the analysis of these ideas and their import herein are accurate, it makes little difference whether they originated "exclusively" in Paris, or else were developed previously or contemporaneously in Edinburgh, Berlin, Vienna, etc. Thus, as Russ Maulitz notes, the claim is not that 'the French were *sui generis*. . . . What Paris did was to offer a particular convergence of tissue emphasis, lots of bodies (though . . . not the first), lots of schools (though not the first), and physical diagnosis.' (personal email communication, September 11, 2012). The seminal analysis of the impact of the Paris School on U.S. physicians is John Harley Warner, *Against the Spirit of the System: The French Impulse in Nineteenth-Century Medicine* (Baltimore, MD: Johns Hopkins University Press, 2003).

6. Nicholas D. Jewson, "The Disappearance of the Sick-Man from Medical Cosmology, 1770–1870," *Sociology* 10, no. 2 (May 1976): 227. Rosenberg terms this essay an "influential, if categorical" effort. Charles E. Rosenberg, "Disease and Social Order in America," in Charles E. Rosenberg, *Explaining Epidemics and Other Studies in the History of Medicine* (Cambridge, UK: Cambridge University Press, 1992), 267.

7. Jewson, "The Disappearance of the Sick Man."

8. Jewson, "The Disappearance of the Sick Man," 229.

9. Martensen, *The Brain Takes Shape*, 13.

10. Lisa Wynne Smith, "'An Account of an Unaccountable Distemper': The Experience of Pain in Early Eighteenth-Century England and France," *Eighteenth-Century Studies* 41, no. 4 (2008): 459–80, quotation on p. 463.

11. Ibid.

12. Ibid.

13. Esther Cohen, "The Animated Pain of the Body," *American Historical Review* 105, no. 1, accessed June 6, 2009, from http://www.historycooperative.org/journals/ahr/105.1/ah000036.html. Cohen expands on these themes in her recent book on the same subject: Esther Cohen, *The Modulated Scream: Pain in Late Medieval Culture* (Chicago, IL: University of Chicago Press, 2010).

14. Ibid.; and Mitchell B. Merback, *The Thief, the Cross, and the Wheel: Pain and the Spectacle of Punishment in Medieval and Renaissance Europe* (Chicago, IL: University of Chicago Press, 1999).

15. Cohen, "The Animated Pain," 6.

16. Ibid., 6–7.

17. A number of recent studies of pain in the early modern era have emphasized the general and easy linkage between concepts of physical and emotional pain. See, e.g., Hannah Newton, *The Sick Child in Early Modern England, 1580–1720* (New York: Oxford University Press 2012); Hannah Newton, "Children's Physic: Medical Perceptions and Treatment of Sick Children in Early Modern England, c. 1580–1720," *Social History of Medicine* 23, no. 3 (2010): 456–74; Jan Frans van Dijkhuizen and Karl A.E. Enenkel, eds., *The Sense of Suffering: Constructions of Physical Pain in Early Modern Culture* (Leiden, Netherlands: Brill, 2008).

18. Smith, "'An Account of an Unaccountable Distemper,'" Silvia de Renzi, "Witnesses of the Body: Medico-Legal Cases in Seventeenth-Century Rome," *Studies in History and Philosophy of Science* 33, no. 2 (June 2002): 219–42; Cohen, "The Animated Pain of the Body"; Cohen, *The Modulated Scream;* Lisa Silverman, *Tortured Subjects: Pain, Truth, and the Body in Early Modern France* (Chicago, IL: University of Chicago Press, 2001); Merback, *The Thief, the Cross, and the Wheel.*

19. Smith, "'An Account of an Unaccountable Distemper,'" 467.

20. Silverman, *Tortured Subjects*, 63.
21. Jewson, "The Disappearance of the Sick Man."
22. Foucault, *The Birth of the Clinic*, 114–15.
23. In England, the Medical Act of 1858 required two years of study in human anatomy as a prerequisite for a license to practice either medicine or surgery. Elizabeth Hurren, "Whose Body is it Anyway?: Trading the Dead Poor, Coroner's Disputes, and the Business of Anatomy at Oxford University, 1885–1929," *Bulletin of the History of Medicine* 82, no. 4 (2008): 775–818.
24. Foucault, *The Birth of the Clinic*, xvi.
25. The concept of flows itself was central to the humoral conception of illness. Alicia Rankin, "Duchess, Heal Thyself," *Bulletin of the History of Medicine* 82, no. 1 (2008): 109–44; Arikha, *Passions & Tempers;* Martensen, *The Brain Takes Shape.*
26. Martensen, *The Brain Takes Shape*, 95.
27. Hurren, "Whose Body is it Anyway?," 792.
28. Ibid., 792–93.
29. See, e.g., Faith Wallis, "Signs and Senses: Diagnosis and Prognosis in Early Medieval Pulse and Urine Texts," *Social History of Medicine* 13, no. 2 (2000): 265–78; Alisha Rankin, "Duchess, Heal Thyself: Elisabeth of Rochlitz and the Patient's Perspective in Early Modern Germany," *Bulletin of the History of Medicine* 82, no. 1 (2008): 109–44; Smith, "'An Account of an Unaccountable Distemper'"; Claudia Stein, "The Meaning of Signs: Diagnosing the French Pox in Early Modern Augsburg," *Bulletin of the History of Medicine* 80, no. 4 (2006): 617–48; Martensen, *The Brain Takes Shape.*
30. Ray, *The History of Pain*, 99.
31. Morris, "An Invisible History of Pain," 193.
32. Ibid.
33. Noémi Tousignant, "Pain and the Pursuit of Objectivity: Pain-Measuring Technologies in the United States c. 1890–1975," (Ph.D. dissertation, McGill University, 2006): 53.
34. Hodgkiss, *From Lesion to Metaphor.*
35. See Silas Weir Mitchell, *Injuries of Nerves and their Consequences* (Philadelphia, PA: J.P. Lippincott & Co., 1872); Wilhelm Heinrich Erb, *Handbook of Electro-Therapeutics* (New York, NY: William Wood & Company, 1883); and Corning, *A Treatise on Headache and Neuralgia,* 2nd ed. Along with Hammond and neurosurgeon W.W. Keen, Mitchell completes the triumvirate most influential in shaping the early history of neurology in the U.S. Of the three, this essay primarily examines Hammond's work on spinal irritation. Yet among them, Mitchell was probably most interested in pain, and he spent a great deal of time caring for and documenting the pain complaints of American Civil War veterans who had undergone amputations. He famously narrated some of their stories in the canonical and pseudonymous short story, "The Mysterious Case of George Dedlow." An ongoing phase of my overall research project delves into Mitchell's work on phantom limb pain as a means of further evaluating the claims issued herein.
36. Ray, *The History of Pain.*
37. Ibid.
38. Ibid., 182–83.
39. James Leonard Corning, *A Treatise on Hysteria and Epilepsy, with Some Concluding Observations on Insomnia* (Detroit, MI: George S. Davis, 1888), 64.
40. Arikha, *Passions & Tempers,* 261.
41. E.g., James Leonard Corning, *A Treatise on Headache and Neuralgia, Including Spinal Irritation and A Disquisition on Normal and Morbid Sleep,* 3rd ed. (New York, NY: E.B. Treat, 1894); William R. Gowers, *Neuralgia: Its*

Etiology, Diagnosis, and Treatment (New York, NY: William Wood & Co., 1890); James Grant Gilchrist, *Surgical Emergencies and Accidents* (Chicago, IL: Duncan Brothers, 1884); and William A. Hammond, *On Certain Conditions of Nervous Derangement* (New York, NY: G.P. Putnam's Sons, 1881).

42. See Ulla Räisänen, Marie-Jet Bekkers, Paula Boddington, Srikant Sarangi, and Angus Clarke, "The Causation of Disease—The Practical and Ethical Consequences of Competing Explanations," *Medicine, Health Care, and Philosophy* 9, no. 3 (December 2006): 293–306; Sylvia N. Tesh, "Miasma and 'Social Factors' in Disease Causality: Lessons from the Nineteenth Century," *Journal of Health Politics, Policy and Law* 20, no. 4 (Winter 1995): 1001–24; Hamlin, "Predisposing Causes"; and Sylvia N. Tesh, *Hidden Arguments: Political Ideology and Disease Prevention Policy* (New Brunswick, NJ: Rutgers University Press, 1988).

43. Corning, *A Treatise on Headache and Neuralgia*, 3rd ed.; and William A. Hammond, *Spinal Irritation* (Detroit, MI: George S. Davis, 1886).

44. Corning, *A Treatise on Headache and Neuralgia*, 3rd ed.

45. Ibid.; Mary Putnam Jacobi, *Essays on Hysteria, Brain Tumor, and Some Other Cases of Nervous Disease* (New York, NY: G.P. Putnam's Sons, 1888); and David Ferrier, *The Localisation of Cerebral Disease: Being the Gulstonian Lectures of the Royal College of Physicians for 1878* (New York, NY: G.P. Putnam's Sons, 1879). For a recent history of Jacobi with an emphasis on her role in the discourse regarding the propriety of women physicians, see Carla Bittel, *Mary Putnam Jacobi and the Politics of Medicine in Nineteenth-Century America* (Chapel Hill, NC: University of North Carolina Press, 2009).

46. Corning, *A Treatise on Headache and Neuralgia*, 2nd ed., 52.

47. Ibid., 53; Corning, *A Treatise on Headache*, 3rd ed., 85.

48. Marcia Meldrum, "A Capsule History of Pain Management," *Journal of the American Medical Association* 290, no. 18 (2003): 2470–75; Hodgkiss, *From Lesion to Metaphor*. Indeed, physicians frequently distinguished between organic and functional disorders, the latter consisting of a cluster of illness complaints for which the structural lesion could not be located. Physicians who subscribed to such a distinction hardly denied the existence of the very complaints that grounded said distinction.

49. *A Calculus of Suffering: Pain, Professionalism and Anesthesia in Nineteenth-Century America* (New York: Columbia University Press, 1985). Famously, part of the reason J. Marion Sims conducted his experiments regarding a surgical intervention for vesicovaginal fistula on African-American slave women was due to his belief that the slaves had much lower sensitivity to pain than his white patients.

50. *Dying in the City of Blues: Sickle Cell Anemia and the Politics of Race and Health* (Chapel Hill: University of North Carolina Press, 2002). Wailoo is also preparing a monograph that addresses the politics of race and health specifically in context of pain. See "The Politics of Pain: Liberal Medicine, Conservative Care and the Governance of Relief in America Since the 1950," 2010 Fielding F. Garrison Lecture, *American Association for the History of Medicine Annual Meeting* (Rochester, MN, April 30, 2010). Wailoo's work represents the seminal historical analysis of politics, racism, and pain in twentieth-century America.

51. Why such cases were regarded by physicians on both sides of the Atlantic Ocean so differently from other kinds of pain complaints is a fascinating and important question, one that the next phase of my current project sets out to examine in more detail.

52. As Surgeon General for the Union during the Civil War, Hammond also directed some of the efforts at sanitarian reforms during the War that presaged the many postbellum public health reforms. Bonnie Ellen Blustein, *Preserve Your Love for Science: Life of William A. Hammond, American Neurologist* (Cambridge, UK: Cambridge University Press, 2002); William A. Hammond, *A Treatise on Hygiene with Special Reference to the Military Service* (Philadelphia, PA: J.B. Lippincott & Co., 1863).

53. Hammond, *Spinal Irritation*, 19.

54. Following Charcot, most nineteenth-century neurologists conceded that indiscernible lesions existed. The issue, however, was always the technical or epistemic inability to see the relevant lesion rather than any doubt as to its actual existence.

55. "The spinal cord is a long organ, and while one part may be the seat of anemia of the posterior columns, the others may be comparatively healthy. It will be shown, however, that the differences in the symptoms as manifested in the various cases which come under notice, are in the main such as result from the fact that different sections of the posterior columns of the cord are the seats of the lesion." Hammond, *Spinal Irritation*, 29.

56. In the few cases in which post-mortem examinations were made, nothing abnormal was found, a circumstance, however, far more compatible with the idea I have expressed than with any other. Ibid., 53.

57. Ibid., 53.

58. "And what is true of the spinal cord is true of other organs of the body. There is not one which may not be the seat of a morbid process in some exceedingly limited part, while the remainder of its tissue presents no evidence of disease. Indeed, the reverse is the exceptional condition." Hammond, *Spinal Irritation*, 57.

59. "From all these points it appears to me that the pathology of spinal irritation is as clearly made out as that of any other disease in which we do not have the opportunity of making post-mortem examinations, or in which, having such opportunities, the lesion remains undiscovered." Ibid., 67–8.

60. Blustein, *Preserve Your Love for Science*.

61. For a number of specific examples, see Goldberg, "Pain Without Lesion."

62. E.g., Putzel; Landon Carter Gray, *A Treatise on Nervous and Mental Diseases* (Philadelphia, PA: Lea Brothers & Co., 1895).

63. Tousignant, "Pain and the Pursuit of Objectivity"; Karen Halttunen "Humanitarianism and the Pornography of Pain in Anglo-American Culture," *American Historical Review* 100, no. 2 (April 1995): 303–34; Elizabeth B. Clark, "'The Sacred Rights of the Weak': Pain, Sympathy, and the Culture of Individual Rights in Antebellum America," *The Journal of American History* 82, no. 2 (September 1995): 463–93; Pernick, *A Calculus of Suffering*; and James C. Turner, *Reckoning with the Beast: Animals, Pain, and Humanity in the Victorian Mind* (Baltimore, MD: Johns Hopkins University Press, 1980).

64. Martensen, *The Brain Takes Shape*, 202.

4 Objectivity, Subjectivity, and Why the History of Pain is Relevant to Its Contemporary Undertreatment

The previous chapter focused on the history of pain not simply because it is worth studying in its own right. Rather, such history also has profound implications for understanding key features of the meaning of pain in American society today, as well as some of the primary reasons for its devastating undertreatment. The specific argument is that American neurologists' nineteenth-century insistence on discerning objective causes for their patients' pain continues to shape attitudes, practices, and beliefs towards pain in the U.S. today, and is a chief factor in its undertreatment.

The idea that objectivity is a critical concept for understanding the contemporary meaning of pain in the U.S. is evident in the fact that virtually any source that addresses the difficulty of treating pain identifies as a principal reason its subjectivity. The common usage tends to suggest that an illness that conveys objective proof of neither its causes nor its effects is difficult to identify and treat. Not coincidentally, so-called subjective illnesses constitute a central part of the family of illnesses social scientists have named "contested diseases." As the name suggests, such illnesses are typically at greater risk of skepticism and suspicion.[1] The subjectivity of most contested illnesses can usefully be contrasted with the apparent objectivity of other diseases. An obvious example is breast cancer, which features solid pathologies that are discernible via objective methods, and many of whose effects (i.e., physiologic changes in body fluids, blood composition, cellular structure, etc.) can be apprehended by objective methods such as laboratory tests and imaging procedures.

But this discussion generally presumes widespread understandings of the concepts of objective and subjective diseases and their effects. What, for example, makes the MRI of the solid tumor objective and the use of the pain scale subjective? That is, what are the criteria for subjectivity and objectivity in context of disease? This chapter concerns itself with these questions. To understand why the subjectivity of pain apparently poses such a problem in American medicine today, it is critical to understand what is meant by terming certain diseases like pain "subjective" and others like breast cancer "objective." A greater understanding of the idea of objectivity and its relevance both to clinical practice in general, and to the meaning of pain in particular, links key ideas from the history of pain to its present undertreatment.

However, contemporary understandings of objectivity did not simply appear fully formed during the twentieth century. Rather, concepts of objectivity have changed quite dramatically over the last four centuries. Notions of objectivity familiar to early modern scientists like Vesalius and Linnaeus would seem strange to contemporary readers. More familiar concepts of objectivity arise in the middle decades of the nineteenth century, the same period that is the subject of Chapter 3's (this volume) analysis of American neurologists' attitudes, practices, and beliefs regarding pain without lesion. The argument is that this overlapping chronology is not coincidence, and this chapter begins the process of connecting, via a brief historical analysis of the concept of objectivity, the history of pain without lesion to the contemporary undertreatment of pain.

OBJECTIVITY AND ITS HISTORIES

Historians of objectivity in the West have documented a number of different concepts of objectivity from the early modern era to the present. One of these, termed "mechanical objectivity," is particularly important to understanding current conceptions, and begins to take hold during the middle decades of the nineteenth century. To highlight the nature of the change, it is necessary to explain briefly what preceded the rise of mechanical objectivity.

Lorraine Daston and Peter Galison's history of objectivity offers perhaps the most thorough analysis of these changes.[2] Given that the power of the visible lesion is one of the central themes in this book, it is significant that Daston and Galison examine scientific atlases as a way of tracing changes in the concept of objectivity over four centuries. The image of the natural object, which of course includes anatomical objects, is thus the central framework for analysis in Daston and Galison's history. They term the form of objectivity that dominated early modern science as "truth-to-nature" objectivity, which differed from later concepts of objectivity in two principal respects: First, truth-to-nature objectivity lionized the subjective influence of the scientific team in producing the images in the atlas. Second, the goal in truth-to-nature objectivity was the depiction of a perfect archetype of the natural object, rather than the maintenance of exact fidelity to the particular specimen under examination.[3]

As to the significance of subjective influence, in early modern scientific atlases, the worth of the illustrations and woodcuts utilized depended on a combination of the artist's skill with the investigator's subjective expertise. The scientific quality of the knowledge was not a function of the investigator's remoteness from the process by which that knowledge was produced; quite the contrary, the specific expertise and training of the investigator was the primary condition upon which the quality of the knowledge was judged. Linnaeus, for example,

> would have dismissed as irresponsible the suggestion that scientific facts should be conveyed without the mediation of the scientist and ridiculed as absurd the notion that the kind of scientific knowledge most worth seeking was that which depended least on the personal traits of the seeker. These later tenets of objectivity, as they were formulated in the mid-nineteenth century, would have contradicted Linnaeus's own sense of scientific mission. Only the keenest and most experienced observer— who had, like Linnaeus, inspected thousands of different specimens— was qualified to distinguish genuine species from mere varieties, to identify the true specific characters imprinted in the plant, and to separate accidental from essential features.[4]

Thus, the scientific epistemology Daston and Galison describe prior to the nineteenth century reflects entirely different notions of truth value than contemporary versions. In the view of Enlightenment atlas makers, "whatever merit their atlases possessed derived precisely from [expert] discernment and from the breadth and depth of experience in their field upon which discernment rested."[5]

As to the interest in universal archetypes, early modern scientists generally did not aim to maintain exact fidelity to the specimen under analysis in the resulting representation. While scientists were well aware that botanical and herbal specimens, for example, displayed all sorts of particular variations and differences, they aimed to capture via the drawing, woodcut, or painting "pure" phenomena, or archetypes that captured all potential forms of the specimen in question.[6] The idea, then, was that only by empirical investigation into thousands of particular specimens could a universal archetype of the object of inquiry be produced. It was these universals that tended to be imaged in scientific atlases of the time.

From these two points, the key insight regarding truth-to-nature objectivity is that it did not prioritize "authentic" depictions and imagery of plants, botanicals, and even human bodies 'just as they appeared in nature.' The value of scientific images was in large part a function of the expertise of the investigator and the skill of the artist in producing an image that demonstrated the archetypal ideal of the natural object.

These two central features of truth-to-nature objectivity likely seem strange to contemporary readers, because more familiar concepts of objectivity tend to take opposing views of the merits (1) of maximizing subjective influence in the scientific process itself, and (2) of intentionally misrepresenting the particular specimen under analysis in the ensuing depiction. The change from the older truth-to-nature model to the more familiar idea of "mechanical" objectivity begins in earnest in the middle decades of the nineteenth century. In contrast to truth-to-nature concepts, the concept of mechanical objectivity tended to privilege knowledge created with minimal subjective interference in the processes of knowledge production. Daston and Galison characterize the demands of mechanical objectivity as a form of self-abnegation, an intentional blinding of the power of one's own subjective gaze, intended to emulate the rigor and automation of the machine: "The observer now aimed to be a machine—to see as if his inner eye of reasoned sight were deliberately blinded."[7]

Accordingly, it is not coincidental that the concept of mechanical objectivity arose concomitant with the development of a number of novel scientific imaging techniques, including photography, lithography, and X-rays. Physicians and scientists of the time lauded the potential of such procedures to capture natural phenomena 'just as they were,' with as little influence of the investigator as possible.[8] Of course, investigators of the time knew full well that their choices and actions exercised great influence on the knowledge produced, but this had little effect on the ideal implied by mechanical objectivity. The ultimate aim was to eliminate, to the maximum extent possible, human influence on scientific knowledge production, and to maintain the utmost fidelity to the exact specimen under consideration.[9]

MECHANICAL OBJECTIVITY, THE HISTORY OF PAIN, AND ITS CONTEMPORARY UNDERTREATMENT

The ethos of mechanical objectivity explains some key changes in late nineteenth-century medical practices. For example, the fact that American roentgenologists at the fin-de-siécle were willing to suffer and die for the sake of seeing the solid tissues and material pathologies of the inner body is itself testament both to the social and cultural significance of the imaging techniques, and to the importance of deploying an automated, mechanical process in the production of scientific and clinical information.[10] Part of the wonder and power of X-rays was the fact that the images they produced did not depend on any anatomical dissection to reveal the solid tissues and material pathologies of the human body.[11] For late nineteenth-century medical science, the critical feature of mechanical objectivity was its emphasis on the importance of permitting the natural objects under investigation to reveal their secrets. The focus of the clinical gaze shifted away from the embodied subject and towards the discrete objects of disease, especially because the latter were amenable to the kinds of quantifiable and mechanical investigations that facilitated the ideal of mechanical objectivity in the nineteenth and twentieth centuries.[12]

Under a mechanical objectivity paradigm, the emphasis on the veridical nature of the natural objects—their capacity to reveal Truth—increases in importance. These objects had to be represented just as they were, with as little subjective interference from the scientists as possible, precisely because the Truth could be discerned via expert observation of the natural object itself. This larger history of objectivity bears significantly on the history of pain without lesion because the American neurologists surveyed in Chapter 3 (this volume) insisted that the key to understanding their patients' suffering rested in discrete, material lesions and pathologies of the nervous system. The Truth of their patients' pain was to be found in the lesions themselves, the natural objects that became invested with immense importance according to the nineteenth-century concept of mechanical objectivity.

LINKS BETWEEN THE HISTORICAL OBJECTIFICATION OF PAIN AND ITS CONTEMPORARY UNDERTREATMENT

The connection between this history and the contemporary undertreatment of pain follows from the increasing emphasis on material discrete "objective" pathologies that could be clinically correlated with the patient's pain. While the body in pain was not ignored during the late nineteenth century, there is little doubt that the emphasis shifted from the embodied, particular subject experiencing the pain to the discrete, material entities that produced the pain. This objectification has come to have profound consequences for the contemporary treatment of pain.

The principal reason such objectification matters is because pain is highly resistant to objectification; by definition my pain is different from your pain.[13] Most types of pain simply cannot be captured by objectifying tools such as lab tests or imaging procedures. Even if the physician can see on an X-ray the compound fracture that is causing the patient's pain, the pain itself is not observed through the X-ray. More problematic are the many varieties of chronic pain that display no visible pathology to which causation may be attributed.

These difficulties are especially significant where modern clinical method is devoted to objectifying the patient's symptoms in order to arrive at a diagnosis and possible therapies. Tracking the nineteenth-century rise of mechanical objectivity, Resnik, Mehm, and Minard note that

> [t]oday's health care professionals use objective methods to develop and confirm diagnoses. . . . These tests allow clinicians to observe, measure, quantify, and compare various anatomical, biochemical, and physical properties, structures, and functions to determine the presence of a specific disease.[14]

Philosopher and psychiatrist Mark Sullivan expressly notes the implication of clinical method for physicians:

> [w]e are taught that real disease can be identified by tissue pathology. . . . In its purest and most essential form, clinical method diagnosis

consists of making the link between symptoms reported by the patient and a lesion observed in the tissue.[15]

This echoes the idea that a key distinction between contested illnesses like pain and uncontested illnesses like (at least some kinds of) cancer turns on the capacity to identify objective causes, here read as material, visible pathologies. Similarly, Sullivan notes that "[i]n the clinicopathologic method, the autopsy reveals the reality of the disease as visible pathology."[16] This method imbues to medicine

> an entirely objective access to diagnosis. It is now possible for the diagnostic process to completely bypass patients' reports of pain or experience of illness. Physicians need no longer rely on patients' knowledge of or candor about their condition, because physicians have a means to go directly to the disease.[17]

Thus, during the nineteenth century, social, political, and cultural forces combined to shape a method that promised to its adherents a way of moving beyond patient self-reports into the objective truths of the body. Roselyne Ray notes that the nineteenth-century physician used the power of the clinicopathologic method to "make independent observations aside from the patient's description" in diagnosing pain.[18] Indeed, William Hammond expressly declares that the patient's report of their own pain is irrelevant if contradicted by an objective clinical sign.[19]

The idea is that the histories of objectivity and pain without lesion provide the historical link to the contemporary undertreatment of pain. One way of understanding this connection is through what Robert Martensen terms "codes of signification built into [biomedicine's] conceptual foundations."[20] These codes parcel out the sick body into discrete solids, solids which, when malformed or pathological, constitute the pure, objective sign of disease that physicians seek.

However, many pain experiences cannot be correlated with any visible pathology or organic insult. If pain cannot be perceived "in the body" as a material pathology, then pain is not amenable to objectification and presents great difficulties for modern clinical method. My argument is that this discordance between the power of the visible in American medicine and the lack of any visible pathology as to many kinds of pain is a primary factor in its undertreatment.

One piece of evidence supporting this characterization of the problem is what anthropologist Jean Jackson identifies as a moral hierarchy of pain.[21] Where the causes of pain can be observed "in the body" through objective, mechanical instrumentation, the moral value assigned to the pain sufferer is higher, and the pain is more likely to be treated adequately. Given that most kinds of chronic pain typically present with no visible pathologies or lesions, it is unsurprising that chronic pain is at the bottom of this hierarchy. As such, Jackson notes that chronic pain sufferers are less likely to receive adequate treatment than sufferers of acute pain secondary to organic insult.[22]

However, even pain experiences that do present with visible causes are problematic for modern medicine. When a heart monitor shows a certain number of beats per minute, the measure literally is a clinical sign of a rapid heartbeat (tachycardia). Yet when the X-ray reveals the compound fracture or the MRI illustrates the solid tumor, the objects depicted are not literally clinical signs of pain. The fractured bone may cause the pain but does not represent the experience of pain in the same way that the rapid heartbeat represents the experience of tachycardia. As such, even so-called 'visible' pain, such as acute pain secondary to organic insult, remains subjective and hence resistant to the objectifying techniques of clinical practice that are firmly rooted in nineteenth-century conceptualizations. Ultimately, the subjective nature of all pain suggests some reasons for thinking that the power of the visible pathology in American culture remains an especially significant source for assessing the meaning of pain.

MIND-BODY DUALISM, PAIN, AND SUBJECTIVITY

As noted above, Jackson's hierarchy of pain is stratified according to a kind of somatic geography: pain whose causes are obviously located "in the body" tends to be treated better and correlates with lower levels of stigma for the sufferer. But what does it mean for pain to be located "in the body"? The implied contrast, of course, is to pain that is located "in the mind," which in turn suggests that modern clinical method incorporates another conceptual problem in the treatment of pain: the mind-body duality.

Though the mind-body distinction has received tremendous criticism, there is reason to believe that it is still deeply ingrained in modern clinical method. Jackson states that "in clinical practice mind/body dualism constantly emerges."[23] Morris notes that the method "impales the patient on the horns of a potent dilemma: either pain has a visible, objective, physical cause, or it is mental, emotional, imaginary, all in your head."[24] However, it is critical to challenge the idea that pain can be 'all in your head.' Howard Fields notes that because pain is modulated by neural phenomena originating in the brain (rather than exclusively originating from the site of organic insult), there is a very real sense in which pain is necessarily 'in one's head.'[25] Pain physician John Loeser observes the absurdity of the notion that pain is 'in the body:' "Does anyone really believe that a tooth is capable of hurting? Or a back?"[26] Loeser is not denying that the pain sufferer can locate the experience of pain to a specific part of the body, but is rather challenging the category mistake that attributes metaphysical claims to phenomenological statements. That is, there is an important distinction between the patient's phenomenological pronouncement that his/her tooth hurts and the invalid metaphysical inference that the pain is wholly contained within the material structure itself (the tooth).

Yet, clinical method encourages the perpetuation of mind-body dualism inasmuch as it suggests that symptoms of disease ought to be confirmed by looking into the physical and chemical composition of the body. Subjective phenomena like pain do not easily fit into this rubric, and this dissonance has had devastating consequences for providers, for pain sufferers, and for caregivers. Indeed, Jackson argues that one reason chronic pain is so problematic is that it "mysteriously straddles the mind-body boundary."[27]

Because the relationship between the mind and the body is so crucial to unpacking the meaning of pain for pain sufferers, caregivers, and providers alike, I turn now to a close analysis of mind-body dualism in context of subjectivity, consciousness, and pain. The history of neurology and neuroscience has occupied much of the analysis thus far because the relationships between brain, mind, and body constitute a key framework for comprehending the meaning of pain. That such dualism remains pervasive among physicians, scientists, and lay persons suggests that it serves as an important lens for understanding the connections between the absence of visible, material pathology and the undertreatment of pain in American society.

NOTES

1. Aside from chronic pain, examples include chronic fatigue syndrome, Gulf War syndrome, and multiple chemical sensitivities syndrome. Debra A. Swoboda, "Negotiating the Diagnostic Uncertainty of Contested Illnesses: Physician Practices and Paradigms," *Health* 12, no. 4 (2008): 453–78; Joseph Dumit, "Illnesses You Have to Fight to Get: Facts as Forces in Uncertain, Emergent Illnesses," *Social Science & Medicine* 62, no. 3 (2006): 577–90.
2. Lorraine Daston and Peter Galison, *Objectivity* (New York: Zone Books, 2007).
3. Ibid., 55–114.
4. Ibid., 59.
5. Ibid., 67.
6. Ibid., 55–105.
7. Ibid., 140.
8. Ibid.; Tal Golan, "The Emergence of the Silent Witness: The Legal and Medical Reception of X-Rays in the United States," *Social Studies of Science* 34, no. 4 (2004): 469–99; Olaf Breidbach, "Representation of the Microcosm— the Claim for Objectivity in 19th Century Scientific Microphotography," *Journal of the History of Biology* 35, no. 2 (2002): 221–50; Daniel S. Goldberg, "Suffering and Death Among Early American Roentgenologists: The Power of Remotely Anatomizing the Living Body in Fin-de-Siècle America," *Bulletin of the History of Medicine* 85, no. 1 (2011): 1–28; Daniel S. Goldberg, "The History of Scientific & Clinical Images in Mid-to-Late 19th c. American Legal Culture: Implications for Contemporary Law & Neuroscience,"

in *Current Legal Issues: Law and Neuroscience,* ed. Michael Freeman (New York: Oxford University Press, 2011), 505–28.

9. Daston and Galison, *Objectivity.*
10. Goldberg, "Suffering and Death"; Goldberg, "The History of Scientific and Clinical Images."
11. Goldberg, "Suffering and Death."
12. See Porter, *Trust in Numbers.*
13. Daniel S. Goldberg, "The Sole Indexicality of Pain: How Attitudes towards the Elderly Erect Barriers to Pain Management," *Michigan State University Journal of Medicine & Law* 12, no. 3 (2008): 51–72; Mark D. Sullivan, "Finding Pain Between Minds and Bodies," *The Clinical Journal of Pain* 17, no. 2 (2001): 151–55; Mark D. Sullivan, "The Problem of Pain in the Clinicopathological Method," *The Clinical Journal of Pain* 14, no. 3 (1998): 197–201; Marja-Liisa Honkasalo, "What is Chronic is Ambiguity: Encountering Biomedicine with Long-Lasting Pain," *Journal of the Finnish Anthropological Society* 24, no. 4 (1999): 79–91; David B. Morris, *Illness and Culture in the Postmodern Age* (Berkeley, CA: University of California Press, 1998), 107–34; David B. Morris, *The Culture of Pain* (Berkeley, CA: University of California Press, 1991); Elaine Scarry, *The Body in Pain: The Making and Unmaking of the World* (New York: Oxford University Press, 1985).
14. David B. Resnik, Marsha Rehm, and Raymond B. Minard, "The Undertreatment of Pain: Scientific, Clinical, Cultural, and Philosophical Factors," *Medicine, Health Care and Philosophy* 4, no. 3 (2001): 282–83.
15. Sullivan, "Finding Pain Between Minds and Bodies," 148.
16. Ibid.
17. Ibid.
18. Roselyne Ray, *The History of Pain* (Cambridge, MA: Harvard University Press, 1993), 99.
19. Hammond notes:

> The fact that the patient denies the existence of [spinal] tenderness should have no weight with the physician. Thus, a young lady consulted me for severe infra-mammary pain, headache, and nausea. I at once suspected spinal irritation, but she declared, in answer to my inquiries, that there was no sign of tenderness anywhere over the spinal column. I insisted, however, on a manual examination, and to her great surprise found three spots that were exceedingly painful to slight pressure.

> William A. Hammond, *On Certain Conditions of Nervous Derangement* (New York: G. P. Putnam's Sons, 1881), 35.

20. Robert L. Martensen, *The Brain Takes Shape: An Early History* (New York, NY: Oxford University Press, 2006), 203. The fact that Martensen develops the framework in analyzing the history of the brain in Western culture adds to its relevance to the history of pain inasmuch as the latter is in its nineteenth-century contexts virtually synonymous with the histories of neurology and neuroscience.
21. Jean E. Jackson, "Stigma, Liminality, and Chronic Pain: Mind-Body Borderlands," *American Ethnologist* 32, no. 3 (2005): 332–53.
22. Ibid.
23. Jean E. Jackson, *Camp Pain: Talking with Chronic Pain Patients* (Philadelphia, PA: University of Pennsylvania Press, 2000), 39.
24. David B. Morris, "An Invisible History of Pain: Early 19th-Century Britain and America," *Clinical Journal of Pain* 14, no. 3 (1998): 194.

25. Howard L. Fields, "Setting the Stage for Pain: Allegorical Tales from Neuroscience," in *Pain and Its Transformations: The Interface of Biology and Culture,* eds. Sarah Coakley and Kay Kaufman Shelemay (Cambridge, MA: Harvard University Press, 2007), 36–61.
26. John Loeser, "What is Chronic Pain?" *Theoretical Medicine and Bioethics* 12, no. 3 (1991): 215.
27. Jackson, "Stigma, Liminality, and Chronic Pain," 343.

Section III
Ethics, Subjectivity, and Pain

5 Mind-Body Dualism, Subjectivity, and Consciousness

INTRODUCTION

Distinctions between mind, body, and soul are ancient in origin, though they took on renewed importance in the early modern era and into the Enlightenment. Descartes is typically perceived as either the primary culprit of mind-body dualism or a potent symbol of its force (hence the frequent references to "Cartesian dualism").[1] Attributing such a crabbed perspective to as complicated and as original a thinker as Descartes is unwise. There is good reason to suspect that Descartes does not deserve the opprobrium heaped upon him. Martensen, while acknowledging that the *cogito* ("I think, therefore I am") grounds some version of mind-body dualism, notes a great many of Descartes's other writings that seem to reject a rigorous distinction between mind and body.[2] Morris goes further and argues that mind-body dualism is not Cartesian in origin, and instead is more properly understood as a creature of the Victorian age.[3]

Defending Descartes is not the point. What is important is to assess the role of mind-body dualism in shaping the meaning of pain in American society. Curiously, the fact that scholars have produced innumerable articles, books, and lectures debunking the duality does not seem to have penetrated all that far into understandings of pain, as pain scholars from fields as diverse as anthropology,[4] sociology,[5] narrative studies,[6] psychiatry,[7] and neuroscience[8] note the vigorous persistence of such dualism.

Moreover, virtually all English-language ethnographies of pain among Western populations state or imply that mind-body dualism is a primary schema for interpreting and understanding pain for illness sufferers, providers, and caregivers alike.[9] As such, any analysis of the meaning of pain that does not account for the continued relevance of mind-body dualism is incomplete. More so, as I will argue in Chapter 7 (this volume), any pain policies that do not incorporate such an understanding have little chance of significant impact.

Unlike prior chapters, in which I synthesized claims and evidence from a variety of authorities and sources, in this chapter, I focus primarily on a close reading of one scholar's analysis. The specific question for this chapter is why does mind-body dualism continue to exert such a pull on American under-standings of pain? As to this question, the most helpful account stems from John Searle's analysis on subjectivity and consciousness.

Before proceeding, it is important to note that this chapter does not of-fer a philosophical analysis of consciousness, which continues to generate vigorous debate in philosophy, psychology, psychiatry, and neuroscience. Yet, Searle's perspective is crucial at least in part because of his notion that the chief flaw in many dominant accounts of mind and consciousness is their failure to proffer an adequate account of subjectivity. The reason that Searle's analysis is so important is the thesis of this book: pain is so poorly treated in the U.S. primarily because the irreducibly subjective phenomenon of pain resists objectification. Pain maps out poorly onto a conception of illness in which visible material pathology occupies pride of place among both illness sufferers and providers.

While Searle is concerned primarily with the role of subjectivity in con-sciousness, it is no accident that so many of his examples and arguments reference pain.[10] The experience of pain features so prominently in Searle's account of consciousness precisely because pain is the quintessentially subjective phenomenon. Accordingly, if subjectivity is central in Searle's account, pain is a particularly instructive case study for thinking about consciousness.

SEARLE'S ACCOUNT OF THE ROLE OF SUBJECTIVITY IN CONSCIOUSNESS

Searle's account of consciousness, explicated primarily through his 1992 monograph, *The Rediscovery of Mind,* and a 2000 essay in the *Annual Reviews of Neuroscience,* begins with his solution to the mind-body prob-lem.[11] This solution is deceptively simple: "Mental phenomena are caused by neurophysiological processes in the brain and are themselves features of the brain."[12] However, as he goes on to explain, they are not reducible to such processes. "The brain causes certain 'mental' phenomena, such as conscious mental states, and these conscious states are simply higher-level features of the brain."[13]

Searle does not regard mental phenomena as composed of a different substance, floating in the ether: "[m]ental events and processes are as much part of our biological natural history as digestion, mitosis, meiosis, or enzyme secretion."[14] He is therefore happy to term himself a "biological naturalis[t],"[15] although he is not a strict biological reductionist. This is because, for Searle, there is more to mind than neurophysiological substrate, even while such substrate is assuredly a *sine qua non* for mind. As such, Searle rejects both dualism and monism. He continually wonders why both positions are deemed to "exhaust the field" such that mind—a term that I will use interchangeably with consciousness[16]—is perceived to be either reducible to neurophysiological substrate *or* to exist in the ether, independent of and not contingent upon such substrate. "The fact that a feature is mental does not imply that it is not physical; the fact that a feature is physical does not imply that it is not mental."[17]

Linking this seemingly ubiquitous reductionism to traditional notions of objectivity, Searle notes that

> [w]e have the conviction that if something is real, it must be equally accessible to all competent observers. Since the seventeenth century, educated people in the West have come to accept an absolutely metaphysical presupposition: Reality is objective. This assumption has proved useful to us in many ways, but it is obviously false, as a moment's reflection on one's own subjective states reveals. And this assumption has led, perhaps inevitably, to the view that the only "scientific" way to study the mind is as a set of objective phenomena. Once we adopt the assumption that anything that is objective must be equally accessible to any observer, the questions are automatically shifted away from the subjectivity of mental states toward the objectivity of the external behavior.[18]

There are a number of important points in this excerpt. First, this is a particular (historical) conception of objectivity—a proposition that *x* is objective if and only if "it is equally accessible to all competent observers."[19] Second, Searle traces this conception to the seventeenth century, which is consistent with my analysis regarding the increasing power of the visible and its link to the clinicopathologic method (though if Daston and Galison are correct, the nineteenth century is significantly more important in framing contemporary notions of objectivity). Third, the notion that only objective phenomena are real in Searle's sense is "obviously false" because one has subjective mental states that by definition are not equally accessible to all. He notes later that "[t]here are lots of empirical facts that are not equally accessible to all observers."[20] As an example, he cites the evidence that birds navigate using the earth's magnetic field:

> It is, I take it, an empirical fact whether or not birds navigate by detecting the magnetic field actually have a conscious experience of the detection of the magnetic field. But the exact qualitative nature of this empirical fact is not accessible to standard forms of empirical tests. And indeed, why should it be? Why should we assume that all the facts in the world are equally accessible to standard, objective, third-person tests? If you think about it, the assumption is obviously false.[21]

Of course, this leaves unanswered an important question related to the ontological status of subjective mental states. If it is the case that we have subjective mental states, and if there are many facts in the world that are not accessible to all competent observers, why is it that a paradigm case of such a state—pain—is doubted because it is not equally accessible to all? This is another way of phrasing the central question of this book.

Fourth, Searle indicates that the notion that reality is objective has led to a belief that the only scientific way to study consciousness is as a set of objective phenomena. Perhaps this explains Amanda Pustilnik's observation that contemporary neuroscientists are often cheerful and committed reductionists.[22] There is therefore some reason to believe that within neuroscience, there is an impetus to reduce mind to brain precisely because the brain can be objectified.[23]

As noted in the previous two chapters, this kind of objectification is fundamentally tied to the nineteenth-century rise of modern clinical method. Accordingly, Searle observes that, in his experience, scientists frequently assert that consciousness is beyond their ken: "The deepest reason for the fear of consciousness is that consciousness has the essentially terrifying feature of subjectivity."[24]

Searle's basic claim is that materialism, roughly defined as the belief that consciousness is reducible to material (neurobiological) substrate, leaves out the crucial role subjectivity plays in constituting consciousness:

> What we find in the history of materialism is a recurring tension between the urge to give an account of reality that leaves out any reference to the special features of the mental, such as consciousness and subjectivity, and at the same time account for our 'intuitions' about the mind.[25]

Again, he emphasizes that there is nothing about the necessity of subjectivity in consciousness that implies that subjective mental states exist independent of neurobiological substrate. Even referring to "subjective mental states" is redundant, because "[m]ental states only exist as subjective, first-person phenomena."[26]

For Searle, the role of subjectivity in consciousness and pain is a function of its first-person status. That is, pain is

> not equally accessible to all observers. . . . For it to be a pain, it must be somebody's pain; and this in a much stronger sense than the sense in which a leg must be somebody's leg, for example. Leg transplants are possible; in that sense, pain transplants are not. And what is true of pain is true of conscious states generally. Every conscious state is always someone's conscious state.[27]

This reference to consciousness in terms of pain, among many others, makes sense because Searle believes that subjectivity is the key element of consciousness. As such, he goes on to explain that subjectivity is inherently "perspectival" in that "[t]he world itself has no point of view, but my access to the world through my conscious states is . . . always from my point of view."[28]

Because pain is perspectival, pain is *necessarily* particular, acculturated, and context-dependent. Pain scholars strongly endorse the idea that cultural and social phenomena are constitutive of pain experience.[29] To link this back to consciousness, Searle reasons that *"If we try to draw a picture of some-one else's consciousness, we just end up drawing the other person* (perhaps with a balloon growing out of his or her head). *If we try to draw our own consciousness, we end up drawing whatever it is that we are conscious of."*[30] This highlights an important feature of consciousness: our own conscious-ness is invisible to us. To argue for this, Searle first suggests that there is no way to observe another's consciousness. Instead, what is observed is "him and his behavior and the relations between him, the behavior, the structure, and the environment."[31]

This seems uncontroversial, but what happens when a person tries to observe his/her own consciousness? Searle answers: "The very fact of subjec-tivity, which we were trying to observe, makes such an observation impos-sible. Why? Because where conscious subjectivity is concerned, there is no distinction between the observation and the thing observed, between the perception and the object perceived."[32] Thus, Searle concludes, "[a]ny intro-spection I have of my own conscious state is itself that conscious state."[33]

Searle's point is that not only are we unable to observe another person's subjectivity, but we also cannot observe our own subjectivity, "for any observation that I might care to make is itself that which was supposed to be observed."[34] If Searle is correct, this again demonstrates the significance of his earlier point that there are many real phenomena in this world that cannot be accessed equally by all observers. This idea can be translated into more concrete terms: the fact that we cannot measure or quantify a phe-nomenon fails to establish that the phenomenon is not real. This argument has important implications for pain, as there is good reason to believe that a primary reason pain is managed so poorly is because it cannot be seen, mea-sured, or quantified "objectively."

REDUCTIONISM, PAIN, AND PHENOMENOLOGY

Searle addresses reductionism in detail, and suggests that what he terms "ontological reductionism" is linked in a scientific context to the general trend "toward greater generality, objectivity, and redefinition in terms of underly-ing causation."[35] Yet, Searle argues, consciousness is irreducible. In demon-strating this, he once again turns to the example of pain:

> Suppose we tried to say the pain is really "nothing but" the patterns of neuron firings. Well, if we tried such an ontological reduction, the essential features of the pain would be left out. No description of the third-person, objective, physiological facts would convey the subjective, first-person character of the pain. . . . [S]omeone who had a complete

knowledge of the neurophysiology of a mental phenomenon such as pain would still not know what a pain was if he or she did not know what it felt like.[36]

A phenomenological approach coheres with Searle's argument here. Akin to Matthews's arguments on the incoherence of conceiving of the lived experience of depression in terms of serotonin levels, it is absurd to claim that the phenomenon of pain is exhausted by patterns of neuron firings. One way of apprehending this apparent absurdity would be to imagine a health care provider informing a patient suffering from intense pain that their conscious experience is equivalent to and is *nothing but* neuronal firing. It is difficult to imagine the pain sufferer who would accept such a claim.

Walter Glannon adduces similar points in an aptly titled article: "Our Brains Are Not Us." Adopting a phenomenological approach, Glannon confirms the emergent, subjective, nonlinear account of mind:

> The mind can be described as a set of unconscious and conscious states that emerge from the brain and its interaction with the body and environment. The mind emerges at a higher level from lower-level brain functions in order to promote the adaptability and survival of the organism within the environment. This cannot be done by neurons, axons, synapses, and neurotransmitters alone. . . . It is not the brain but the subject constituted by the brain and the mind who is the agent.[37]

Searle elucidates this point further by explaining how the objectification utilized in the scientific and clinical gaze is unable to account for the subjective experiences of pain and consciousness:

> We could simply define, for example, "pain" as patterns of neuronal activity that cause subjective sensations of pain. And if such a redefinition took place, we would have achieved the same sort of reduction for pain that we have for heat. But of course the reduction of pain to its physical reality still leaves the subjective experience of pain unreduced, just as the reduction of heat left the subjective experience of heat unreduced.[38]

The idea here is not that the neurobiological causes of pain are somehow disconnected or irrelevant to the experience of pain, but that the experience of pain as a phenomenon is simply not reducible to neurobiology. Searle continues:

> Part of the point of the reductions was to carve off the subjective experiences and exclude them from the definition of the real phenomena, which are now defined in terms of those features that interest us most.

But where the phenomena that interest us most are the subjective experiences themselves, there is no way to carve anything off.[39]

In other words, whether the phenomenon in question is consciousness or its manifestation as pain, it is precisely those subjective, first-person experiences that matter. This has important ramifications for the efforts to obtain objective evidence of pain. If what we are "interested in" is irreducibly subjective, then any effort to objectify pain is incoherent. It is, to borrow my favorite metaphor of Wittgenstein's, an attempt to open doors that are painted on to walls.[40] What we might like to know most about pain is precisely what we can never capture objectively, because any objective measure by definition tells us nothing about the subjective phenomenon of pain. Resnik, Rehm, and Minard concur, arguing that such attempts are chimerical:

> [P]ain assessment tools will never achieve the degree of objectivity that one finds in most medical tests, since pain will still be a subjective sensation or feeling. . . . We can no more test for pain than we can test for a person's enjoyment of Mozart, distaste for anchovies, or fear of the IRS.[41]

But, one could object to this claim by arguing that we can use novel neuroimaging techniques to test for a person's enjoyment of Mozart, distaste for anchovies, or fear of the IRS. And if we can do so, why could the same kind of neuroimaging techniques not be used to show pain, to render it finally visible and objective?

PAIN, SUBJECTIVITY, AND NEUROREDUCTIONISM

The hypothetical study would follow the standard fMRI protocol. Baseline readings would be taken of a subject, followed by application of the stimulus and comparison of blood oxygenation levels in the relevant (read: localized) region of the brain. If the observed activation levels reach the desired measure of significance, then the study has presumably identified a neural correlate of "enjoying Mozart." Indeed, one such study, entitled "A Functional MRI Study of Happy and Sad Affective States Induced by Classical Music," has already been published.[42]

However beguiling, such an argument is what Racine, Bar-Ilan, and Illes have referred to as the fallacy of "neuro-realism."[43] It is the same category mistake referenced in Loeser's challenge ("Does anyone really think that a tooth is capable of hurting? Or a back?"). The idea that quantifying blood oxygenation levels literally captures the experience of "enjoying Mozart" is absurd. The very terminology used in the neuroimaging literature demonstrates this, as the phrase "neural correlate" implies that the analysis merely attempts to correlate a particular function with increased blood oxygenation. The conclusion that the experience of pain is reducible to such increased blood oxygenation is both absurd and false. Glannon concurs, noting that the claim is erroneous even on its own terms, because such images "are visualizations of statistical analyses based on large numbers of images and are more accurately described as scientific constructs than actual images of the brain."[44] But, he continues, "[e]ven if imaging could tell us what actually occurred in the brain," the category error still vitiates the claim: "it could not tell us what actually occurred in the brain, it could not reproduce the phenomenological feel of what it is like for a subject to experience events in the world."[45]

In short, there is no conceivable sense in which any method of objectification could entirely account for the irreducibly subjective phenomenon of pain. This is not to suggest that it is mistaken to argue that patterns of neuronal firing are a necessary cause for pain. Searle's point is precisely that such neurophysiological phenomena are indeed such a cause of pain, but that this causal account alone is insufficient to capture the phenomena of pain. Similarly, the argument is not that objectifying modalities have no place in diagnosing and treating pain, but rather that the notion that neuroimaging techniques can characterize what the experience of pain is like for the pain sufferer is dangerously misguided. Searle therefore concludes that the "antireductionist argument . . . is ludicrously simple and quite decisive."[46]

However, if this is so, why are such neurofallacies so common? Why do so many scholars and lay people suggest that neuroimaging techniques provide objective evidence of that which cannot be objectified (pain)? Perhaps more to the point, why do we perpetually seek to objectify that which cannot be objectified?

One answer emphasizes the hold that seeing inside the body and, in particular, seeing inside the brain exerts in American society.[47] These scientific and clinical images bestow the power to make pain real, and, as such, it is unsurprising to see the effects of such dualism pervading the meaning-making endeavors of chronic pain sufferers themselves.

PAIN SUFFERERS, MIND-BODY DUALISM, AND THE POWER OF IMAGING

The convergence between the power of the visible and mind-body dualism for pain sufferers in the U.S. is powerfully demonstrated in Rhodes, McPhillips-Tangum, Markham, and Klenk's 1999 study, aptly entitled "The Power of the Visible: The Meaning of Diagnostic Tests in Chronic Back Pain."[48] Chronic back pain is an especially significant choice for analysis because, as illustrated in Chapter 1 (this volume), chronic back pain is both particularly prevalent in the U.S., and back pain treatments are frequently ineffective and unsatisfying for patients.[49] Moreover, chronic back pain often presents with no evidence of visible, material pathologies.[50]

One theme that emerges from Rhodes, McPhillips-Tangum, Markham, and Klenk's study is the concreteness promised by imaging tests: "They call on the patient to align herself with their reality, demanding to be read as factual evidence of a match between the inside of the body as 'specimen' and the inside of the body as the private and incontrovertible ground of experience."[51] The suggestion that the images of the inner body produced by imaging techniques are deemed to be real echoes both Searle's analysis on the "reality" of objectivity and my argument regarding the relationship between internal pathologies and external signs or symptoms.

The concreteness of visible images of the material structures of the inner body is closely tied with the themes of legitimacy and justification:

> Patients for whom something 'shows' on tests emphasize a feeling of justification, of not being 'crazy.' Tests 'show where it hurts' and confirm the reality of pain: in fact, patients repeatedly use the word real to describe this confirmation and remark that what 'shows' is 'obvious' and 'concrete.'[52]

This passage underscores several important points. First, what is most significant for the pain sufferers is what *shows* via diagnostic imaging tests. The power of the visible in making meaning of pain is therefore not limited solely to providers, but is a primary narrative for pain sufferers themselves. Jackson writes of one pain sufferer's frustration with the inability of his physicians to produce visible images of the cause of his pain: "He would go for tests hoping fervently that something would show up, and after a while he did not care what it was."[53] Second, the imaging tests enable localization of pain, they "show where it hurts." Chapters 3 and 4 (this volume) show that the significance of localizing pain extends at least as far back as the nineteenth century, and is tied to the importance of identifying visible, material pathologies as the seat of pain. Moreover, pain sufferers as well as providers connect the legitimacy and reality of pain to its localizability.

Honkasalo notes that the chronic pain sufferers in her ethnography tended to localize their pain: "In her story, Anniki said that the pain 'usually lives in her left hip, loin and thigh.' 'Often it is so circumscribed that I feel, if it could be surgically removed, I'd be healthy.' The strict localization affirmed her thoughts about the biomedical etiology of her pain."[54] Honkasalo thus connects the meaning-making power of the localization of pain to mind-body dualism. Such localization is crucial to the pain sufferers precisely because it indicates that the seat of the pain is *in the body*. However, as I have argued throughout this book, the notion of a distinction between pain that is "in the body" and pain that is "in the mind" is incoherent, because cognitive and affective processes are inextricably linked to pain. Fields's point is precisely that the neurobiology of pain cannot be separated from the meaning of pain, because our ways of understanding pain alter neurochemical pathways and vice-versa in the circular feedback loop patterns characteristic of complex adaptive systems.[55] Thus, he notes, "all pain is mental."[56]

But the incoherence of this distinction belies its persistence among lay persons and providers; pain that is localizable in the body via imaging techniques makes otherwise invisible pain real. Without visible images demonstrating the seat of the pain in visible, material pathologies, pain sufferers themselves doubt the legitimacy of their pain. So powerful is the reifying potential of seeing the visible material pathologies that cause their pain that some pain sufferers in the Rhodes et al. study express palpable relief when anomalies show up on imaging tests, even when such anomalies portend invasive surgeries:

> In an instant [the] patient goes from feeling disbelieved—that she has to 'insist' in the face of repeated disappointment—to an intense feeling of relief, despite the fact that what has been found means that she faces surgery. What she had been saying to her doctor could not be heard until, to her joy, it could be seen. Patients who describe events like this express satisfaction even when the diagnosis itself does not suggest imminent or even eventual relief.[57]

The second sentence in this quotation—the difference between voicing complaints that were not heard and seeing causes of signs and symptoms—exactly tracks Foucault's depiction of the changes between eighteenth-century and nineteenth-century medical cosmologies (the difference between the questions 'what is the matter with you' and 'where does it hurt'). The meaning made in seeing the visible, material pathologies that cause the pain is such that even the prospect of invasive, presumably painful surgeries on the pain sufferer's back is of comparatively less significance.

Both of the pain sufferers whom the authors describe ("Pam" and "Stan")

> emphasize that the role of the doctor is to *look*. Pam describes her doctor as 'willing to look' and Stan expresses frustration that his does not look farther. . . . He persists in believing that his doctors *can not* have run all the tests if his back still hurts.[58]

The physician's role in constructing a meaningful story with the patient[59] centers on the physician's ability to find the visible, material causes of the patient's suffering. This is why, in Honkasalo's study, one sufferer, "Anniki," bore a grudge against physicians "because they did not find any special causal agent."[60] Tracking the importance of localization and mind-body dualism I have addressed, Stan cannot account for the persistence of his pain if no test or objective procedure can image it; its correspondence with 'reality' is diminished in the absence of the ability to see.

Thus, the meaning-making power of the clinical gaze is not only a phenomenon providers attempt to harness, but is also a narrative that pain sufferers, often desperate for validation and relief, return to as well: "Diagnostic testing holds out the possibility that they can *see* where deviation occurs and despite their expressions of hostility, they live in the same universe of explanation as their doctors."[61]

Jackson's observations are consistent with the Rhodes et al. study, and she notes that "I collected many statements from both patients and staff members characterizing 'real' pain in this way—real because one can see it on an X-ray, CT scan, or blood test."[62] Jackson uses even stronger language to explain the collaborative dynamic that providers and pain sufferers use to make meaning of the pain: "With few exceptions, medical practitioners and patients in pain generally collude to maintain a conceptual separation between the mind and the body and search for objective evidence of an underlying organic condition."[63] The pain patients Jackson studied desperately searched for "validation of their pain" and "tended to rely on any available objective measure that made their pain as 'real' as possible."[64] In a grotesque irony, the power of mind-body dualism is such that chronic pain sufferers—who often have their pain delegitimized and invalidated—join providers in the search for objective evidence of their pain, even while that very search contributes to the invalidation and denial of the reality of their pain.

I am certainly not blaming pain sufferers for employing meaning-making strategies in the face of pain that serve to strengthen the social and cultural dynamics that animate the general stigmatization and undertreatment of pain. Many pain sufferers are desperate in a variety of ways. Even assuming the best of intentions from providers and caregivers, the evidence suggests that pain sufferers are often stigmatized, are often not heard, and frequently have their experiences invalidated and delegitimized.[65] In addition to these problems, many pain sufferers do just that—they suffer, and they often experience great difficulty in making meaning of their pain. There is no rationale for faulting pain sufferers for seeking narratives, which, by virtue of their social and cultural significance, seem to provide ways of relieving their desperation and making meaning of their suffering.

The point of the analysis is to explain how and why pain sufferers do conceptualize and understand their own pain in very similar frames as do their providers, and to argue that the emphasis on and power of the visible animates a conceptual scheme in which lay and professional are both active participants. The idea is not that pain sufferers should be blamed for seeking the power of imaging tests or mind-body dualism in making sense of pain; rather, the key idea is that they *do* understand and conceptualize their own pain experiences according to such frames. Ultimately, as I will argue in Chapter 8 (this volume), any legitimate pain policies must account for these deep-seeded ways of understanding the meaning of pain.

CONCLUSION

The primary aim of this chapter was to articulate and defend Searle's account of consciousness, which prominently features an irreducible, unquantifable subjectivity. Such an account eschews mind-body dualism, accepting neither that consciousness is reducible to neurophysiological substrate nor that consciousness is possible in the absence of such substrate. Consciousness is emergent, arising from biochemical, physiological, and environmental (social and cultural) interactions and pathways, but reducible to none of these constituent parts.

This account has profound implications for understanding the meaning of pain in American society. It grounds the prevailing view that pain is quintessentially subjective, and demonstrates the mistakes of conception and practice that attend the constant efforts to "carve out" or excise subjective elements from objects of inquiry (such as "pain" or "consciousness"). Unfortunately, Searle correctly notes that such efforts are common components of Western science and medicine, at least since the early modern era, and especially since the nineteenth century. Subjective phenomena that are not perceptible in visible, material pathologies inside the body are invisible to the clinical gaze, and, as such, are subject to grave doubts as to their reality and legitimacy. Furthermore, such doubts underscore the persistent and powerful grip mind-body dualism continues to exert on both lay and professional conceptions of health, illness, and pain.

This dynamic of doubt is so powerful that pain sufferers internalize it, desperately seeking visible "proof" of the pathologies understood to be causing or at least correlated with their chronic pain. The pain sufferers participate, or "collude," to use Jackson's term, in the very process of seeking to objectify that which defies objectification. Sadly, however, pain sufferers do not have the luxury of doubting the lived experience of their own pain, even while their attempts to objectify their pain merely reinforce the conceptual categories that facilitate the stigmatization so many pain sufferers experience.

NOTES

1. E.g., Antonio R. Damasio, *Descartes' Error: Emotion, Reason, and the Human Brain* (New York: Quill, 1994).
2. Martensen, *The Brain Takes Shape*, 47–75, 129–34, 209–13.
3. Morris, "An Invisible History of Pain"; Morris, *The Culture of Pain*. See also Grant Duncan, "Mind-Body Dualism and the Biopsychosocial Model of Pain: What Did Descartes Really Say?" *Journal of Medicine and Philosophy* 25, no. 4 (2000): 485–513.
4. E.g., Jackson, "Stigma and Chronic Pain."
5. E.g., Gillian A. Bendelow and Simon J. Williams, "Transcending the Dualisms: Towards a Sociology of Pain," *Sociology of Health & Illness* 17, no. 2 (March 1995): 139–65.

6. E.g., Morris, "An Invisible History of Pain"; Morris, *The Culture of Pain.*
7. E.g., Sullivan, "Finding Pain Between Minds and Bodies."
8. E.g., Fields, "Setting the Stage for Pain."
9. E.g., Jackson, "Stigma, Liminality, and Chronic Pain"; Susan Greenhalgh, *Under the Medical Gaze: Facts and Fictions of Chronic Pain* (Berkeley, CA: University of California Press, 2001); Jackson, *Camp Pain;* Honkasalo, "Chronic Pain as a Posture"; Honkasalo, "What is Chronic is Ambiguity"; Bendelow and Williams, "Transcending the Dualisms"; Arthur Kleinman, "Pain as Resistance: The Delegitimation and Relegitimation of Social Worlds," in *Pain as Human Experience,* eds. Paul E. Brodwin, Arthur Kleinman, Byron J. Good, and Mary-Jo DelVecchio Good (Berkeley, CA: University of California Press, 1992), 169–97; Jackson, "'After a While, No One Believes You'"; Joseph A. Kotarba, *Chronic Pain: Its Social Dimensions* (Beverly Hills, CA: Sage Publications, 1983); Mark Zborowski, *People in Pain* (San Francisco, CA: Jossey-Bass, 1969); Mark Zborowski, "Cultural Components in Responses to Pain," *Journal of Social Issues* 8, no. 4 (1952): 16–30.
10. Indeed, reference to pain is commonplace among philosophical treatments of consciousness. I will elucidate the reasons for this below.
11. Searle develops his account at length in the *Rediscovery of Mind,* and as such I will focus almost exclusively on this text. There is no indication in the 2000 essay or in any other of Searle's writings that he has significantly changed his views on the role of subjectivity in consciousness.
12. John Searle, *The Rediscovery of Mind* (Cambridge, MA: The MIT Press, 1992), 1.
13. Ibid., 14.
14. Ibid., 1.
15. Ibid.
16. This is not to assume that "mind" and "consciousness" are identical, but merely that whatever difference exists between the two terms is immaterial to the purposes for which I use them.
17. Ibid., 14–15.
18. Ibid., 16.
19. Ibid.
20. Ibid., 72.
21. Ibid., 73.
22. Pustilnik, "Violence on the Brain"; see also Joelle M. Abi-Rached and Nikolas Rose, "The Birth of the Neuromolecular Gaze," *History of the Human Sciences* 23, no. 1 (2010): 11–36; Walter Glannon, "Our Brains Are Not Us," *Bioethics* 23, no. 6 (July 2009): 321–9.
23. In her account of the various attempts to measure and objectify pain in the United States during the twentieth century, Noèmi Tousignant confirms just such a suspicion. Tousignant documents how the dolorimeter, popularized during the 1940s and 1950s, fell out of favor among scientists and physicians precisely because it failed to produce consistent, replicable, objective data regarding clinical pain. In his pioneering of the analgesic clinical trial during the 1950s and 1960s, Henry Beecher successfully undermined prevailing medical and scientific acceptance of the dolorimeter in large part because he showed that the analgesic clinical trial could better objectify clinical pain. This suggests that the preference for a particular means of measuring pain reflects attitudes, practices, and beliefs regarding what features of the phenomenon of pain are most significant. The success of the analgesic clinical trial illustrates that the focus on objectification and aggregation of pain experiences received the lion's share of the attention and resources directed to pain during the middle decades of the twentieth century. See Noèmi

Tousignant, "The Rise and Fall of the Dolorimeter: Pain, Analgesics, and the Management of Subjectivity in Mid-twentieth-Century United States," *Journal of the History of Medicine and Allied Sciences* 66, no. 2 (2010): 145–79; Tousignant, "Pain and Objectivity." On the role of quantification in the history of objectivity, see Theodore M. Porter, *Trust in Numbers: The Pursuit of Objectivity in Science and Public Life* (Princeton, NJ: Princeton University Press, 1995); and Peter Dear, "From Truth to Disinterestedness in the Seventeenth Century," *Social Studies of Science* 22, no. 4 (November 1992): 619–31.

24. Searle, *The Rediscovery of Mind*, 55.
25. Ibid., 52.
26. Ibid., 70.
27. Ibid., 94–5.
28. Ibid., 95.
29. Fields, "Setting the Stage for Pain," Laurence Kirmayer, "On the Cultural Mediation of Pain," in *Pain and Its Transformations: The Interface of Biology and Culture*, eds. Sarah Coakley and Kay Kaufman Shelemay (Cambridge, MA: Harvard University Press, 2007), 363–401; Jackson, "Stigma, Liminality, and Chronic Pain"; Jackson, *Camp Pain*; Morris, *The Culture of Pain*.
30. Searle, *The Rediscovery of Mind*, 96 (emphases in original).
31. Ibid., 97.
32. Ibid.
33. Ibid.
34. Ibid., 99.
35. Ibid., 116.
36. Ibid., 117–18.
37. Glannon, "Our Brains are Not Us," 322.
38. Searle, *The Rediscovery of Mind*, 121.
39. Ibid.
40. Douglas A. Gasking and Alan C. Jackson, "Wittgenstein as a Teacher," in *Ludwig Wittgenstein: The Man and his Philosophy*, ed. Kenneth T. Fann (New York, NY: Humanities Press 1978), 169–83.
41. Resnik, Rehm, and Minard, "The Undertreatment of Pain," 284.
42. Martina T. Mitterschiffthaler, Cynthia H. Y. Fu, Jeffrey A. Dalton, Christopher M. Andrew, and Steven C. R. Williams, "A Functional MRI Study of Happy and Sad Affective States Induced by Classical Music," *Human Brain Mapping* 28, no. 11 (November 2007): 1150–62.
43. Eric Racine, Ofek Bar-Ilan, and Judy Illes, "fMRI in the Public Eye," *Nature Reviews Neuroscience* 6, no. 2 (2005): 159–64.
44. Glannon, "Our Brains Are Not Us," 325. See also Vul, Harris, Winkielman, and Pashler, "Puzzlingly High Correlations in fMRI Studies"; Kelly Joyce, *Magnetic Appeal: MRI and the Myth of Transparency* (Ithaca, NY: Cornell University Press, 2008); Kelly Joyce, "Appealing Images: Magnetic Resonance Imaging and the Production of Authoritative Knowledge," *Social Studies of Science* 35, no. 3 (June 2005): 437–62; and Joseph Dumit, *Picturing Personhood: Brain Scans and Biomedical Identity* (Princeton, NJ: Princeton University Press, 2003).
45. Glannon, "Our Brains Are Not Us," 325.
46. Searle, *The Rediscovery of Mind*, 118.
47. See Dumit, *Picturing Personhood*.
48. Rhodes, McPhillips-Tangum, Markham, and Klenk, "The Power of the Visible."
49. William Hammond's treatise on spinal irritation, among many others, suggests that the difficulties in diagnosing and treating chronic back pain are not simply a contemporary problem.

50. John M.S. Pearce, "Chronic Regional Pain and Chronic Pain Syndromes," *Spinal Cord* 43, no. 5 (May 2005): 263–8.
51. Rhodes, McPhillips-Tangum, Markham, and Klenk, "The Power of the Visible," 1193.
52. Ibid., 1194.
53. Jackson, *Camp Pain*, 41.
54. Honkasalo, "Chronic Pain as Posture," 202.
55. Fields, "Setting the Stage for Pain," 36; Glannon, "Our Brains Are Not Us," 328; Newell 2001, "A Theory of Interdisciplinary Studies."
56. Fields, "Setting the Stage for Pain," 36.
57. Rhodes, McPhillips-Tangum, Markham, and Klenk, "The Power of the Visible," 1195.
58. Ibid., 1200 (emphases in original).
59. Brody, *Stories of Sickness*.
60. Honkasalo, "Chronic Pain as Posture," 202.
61. Rhodes, McPhillips-Tangum, Markham, and Klenk, "The Power of the Visible," 1200.
62. Jackson, *Camp Pain*, 148.
63. Ibid., 39.
64. Ibid., 148.
65. Jackson, "Stigma, Liminality, and Chronic Pain."

6 Pain, Objectivity, and Bioethics

INTRODUCTION

Given the power of science and medicine in justifying knowledge claims in the West and the U.S., it is unsurprising that dominant categories of understanding in science and medicine have shaped philosophical discourse. Particularly within moral philosophy, objectivism and realism dominate contemporary work. John Leslie Mackie concurs, observing that "the main tradition of European moral philosophy includes the . . . claim that there are objective values. . . ."[1] This observation certainly applies to traditionally dominant conceptions of bioethics, or at least in the convention in bioethics referred to as principlism.

In this chapter, I have two aims. First, I want to describe principlism and objectivism as it tends to function in bioethics scholarship, and to note some of the critiques of principlist bioethics that have sprung up largely within the last decade. Second, building on these critiques, I will explain how attention to the phenomenology of illness is, unlike principlist bioethics, well-suited to accounting for the ethics of pain. In Chapter 2 (this volume) I explained the features of the phenomenology of pain, but I expressly reserved discussion of the implications of such an account for the ethics of pain. I will assess these implications in this chapter.

Principlism in morals generally refers to the notion that a stock of principles are necessary to account for moral reasoning and moral deliberation, and to guide action. While principlism in bioethics has come under significant attack in the recent decade, reliance on principles has deep roots in the Western ethical tradition, from Plato to Kant to Rawls.

It is therefore important to delineate the narrow scope of my aims in this chapter. It is not intended as a general critique per se of the use of principles in moral thought, but rather as an assessment of why a particular and dominant account of the role of principles in applied ethics is ill-suited for giving ethical account of the body in pain. I make no claims that reliance on principles is inadvisable in all given ethical contexts, nor do I claim that it is impossible to enrich some of the dominant conceptions of principles in bioethics discourse.[2] What I am concerned with in this chapter is a specific discourse and way of practice within bioethics related to the operation and function of principles. I acknowledge the possibility that an objectivist, principle-based ethical approach could in theory illuminate some important features of the ethics of pain; my argument here is simply that the specific versions that have tended to dominate American bioethics practice and scholarship are unhelpful in either assessing the ethical implications of pain or in producing ethical pain policy.

THE ROLE OF PRINCIPLISM IN BIOETHICS

Within bioethics, the most obvious example of the influence of principlism is the aptly titled *Principles of Biomedical Ethics*, authored by Tom Beauchamp and James Childress.[3] First published in 1980, and currently in its sixth edition, the text adopts an overtly principlist approach, generally arguing that four universal principles are most helpful in illuminating bioethics practice: autonomy, beneficence, nonmaleficence, and justice. The text has undergone major changes over the past quarter-century, in no small part because of the merits of the various criticisms that have been launched against it.

Nevertheless, there is little question that Beauchamp and Childress remain committed principlists, and the influence of the textbook suggests how principlism and bioethics have been linked at a deep level almost from the inception of the field of inquiry.[4] Oonagh Corrigan, for example, documents the ways in which a principle-based conception dominates contemporary understandings of informed consent.[5] John Evans suggests that "principlism itself has become an institution."[6] In the sociology of knowledge, Evans explains, an "institution" is defined as "organized, established procedure[s] . . . [which] have taken on a life of their own, independent of the social conditions of their founding, and are self-replicating."[7] He uses the example of Congress, which was presumably intended as a set of organized, established procedures, but which now is "self-replicating and self-justifying," and which "exists independent of the original impetus for its creation. . . ."[8] Principlism, he argues, has similarly taken on a life of its own, though its usage continues to be facilitated by governmental and bureaucratic "appetite[s]" for bioethical decisions."[9]

Moreover, Evans notes that the definition of a "profession" in sociological terms is the maintenance of a "distinct system of knowledge [the profession uses] to solve the problems in [its] jurisdiction. This system is taught by the elite to the average members of the profession—and the dominant system in bioethics is principlism."[10] This is not to imply any false uniformity in bioethics discourse or practice; as we shall see, quite a few scholars and practitioners object to principlism. Rather, the point is that principlism in bioethics has been and continues to be a dominant framework utilized in bioethics practice and discourse, and that, while its dominance hardly goes unchallenged, such challenges are much more likely to come from within the field than from without. Evans concurs: "[T]he average member of an ethics committee is unlikely to question the system—who has the time?—and is going to open his or her copy of Beauchamp and Childress because it sets out a legitimate method for making decisions."[11]

However, what Leigh Turner refers to as the "common morality presumption"[12] is not limited to self-identified principlists within bioethics scholarship, as casuists, common morality proponents such as Bernard Gert, and theorists drawing on the Rawlsian notion of reflective equilibrium all seem to rely on the notion of a universal, common morality. Jonathan Dancy, one of the chief exponents of moral particularism, suggests that inasmuch as all would be comfortable being identified as "moral generalists," they all seem to rely to a greater or lesser extent on principles. Indeed, Dancy expressly links generalism in morals to principlism by defining moral generalism as the notion that "the very possibility of moral thought and judgment depends on the provision of a suitable supply of moral principles."[13]

Regardless of the extent to which moral principlists identify with casuists, common morality proponents, or reflective equilibrium theorists, one characteristic many of these approaches have in common is that they are objectivist in nature. By this I mean that these approaches, which have traditionally dominated both bioethics discourse and practice, tend to presume that morality is metaphysically objective, that there exists a notion of morality that does not depend for its rightness or wrongness on any subjective states or propositions. For the moral objectivist, the fact that a moral agent deems abortion to be immoral does not in and of itself suffice to establish the immorality of abortion. This is because the moral objectivist maintains that there exists an objective, mind-independent morality that does not depend on any moral agent's beliefs about ethics. Admittedly, this proposition seems highly intuitive, which may help explain the "dominance of the objectivist tradition" in moral philosophy.[14]

Mackie notes further that the assumption that "ordinary moral judgments include a claim to objectivity . . . has been incorporated in the basic, conventional meaning of moral terms."[15] Indeed, in his defense of moral objectivism, Justin Felux states that because moral skeptics and anti-realists "are presenting a metaethical system that is very counter-intuitive and defies common sense," it is they who bear the burden of proof.[16]

Felux defines moral objectivism as the thesis that "at least some of our moral judgments are objectively true or false, and that they are true or false regardless of the beliefs or feelings of any particular person or group about them."[17] He acknowledges that "our ethical judgments are both context-dependent and subject-dependent,"[18] but nevertheless argues that propositions such as "It is wrong to punish someone for a crime she did not commit" and "Genocide is wrong" constitute objective moral statements.

His argument for this conclusion rests on a version of moral intuitionism in which the chain of reasoning flows as follows:

1. There are moral propositions.
2. Propositions are either true or false (Law of Excluded Middle).
3. They are not all false.
4. Some correspond to reality (from (2), (3), and the correspondence theory of truth).
5. Moral values are a part of reality (which is moral objectivism).[19]

In contrast, some, like Mackie, contend that "[t]here are no objective values," and that subjectivism in morals overlaps substantially with skepticism in morals.[20] Mackie quickly dispenses with the straw man argument that moral subjectivism constitutes a wholesale rejection of morality; he readily concedes, as do most moral subjectivists, that what he terms "first order normative moral views" do exist. Moreover, he does not assert a first-order claim such as "that everyone really ought to do whatever he thinks he should."[21] Mackie, like Turner and Dancy, is making a metaethical claim, an argument that accounts for a kind of embodied, contextualized sense of the way in which humans tend to utilize moral frameworks in practice.

In *The Moral Imagination*, Mark Johnson terms the dominant conception of Western ethics the "Moral Law Folk Theory." Central to this theory is the presumed existence of "general laws given by universal human reasons concerning which acts we *must* do (prescriptions), which acts we *must not* do (prohibitions), and which acts we *may do*, if we so choose (permissible acts)."[22] While not identical to the rough conception of generalism and principlism that I am working with, I submit there is enough of a family resemblance between Johnson's heuristic and generalism and principlism to make his analysis useful. Johnson does not deny the existence of moral rules, and acknowledges that, "[a]s accretions of the moral wisdom of a tradition or culture, moral rules can serve as summaries of the experience of a people. But it does not follow at all from this that acting morally is reducible to acting in strict accordance with a system of rationally derived rules."[23]

In any case, the overlapping concepts of objectivism, generalism, and realism in morals present complicated, difficult terrain that cannot be fully explicated in an account centered on the subject in pain. I nevertheless maintain that there exists enough meat on the bones to sketch the key point: within Western moral philosophy in general and American bioethics in particular, belief in some version of moral generalism and/or moral principlism has been and remains central.

CRITICISMS OF MORAL PRINCIPLISM

At this point, critiques of the dominance of principlism in bioethics are not new. Many of the most compelling criticisms center on a notion of ethics informed by social science research. For example, Leigh Turner argues that the common morality proponents "simply do not provide the comparative and historical research that might begin to support the argument for the existence of common moral norms found in all societies throughout history."[24] Moreover, he contends, such evidence does not exist:

> [S]cholarship in social history and cultural anthropology attests to the remarkable malleability of communal understandings of morality. The plasticity of understandings of morality across cultures and through time suggests grounds for skepticism concerning the development of a transcultural basis for cross-cultural moral norms. . . . "Human nature" or some shared, cross-cultural sense of moral intuitions does not seem to be a particularly reliable basis upon which to build universalist models of the common morality.[25]

The idea is that the common morality position seems empirically dubious given what we know about cultural relativism, namely, that different communities and societies often have widely variant conceptions of morality. Turner suggests that what he terms moral pluralists "pose the greatest challenge to the common morality approach, because the moral pluralists insist that careful comparative and historical research reveals considerable variability in what constitutes 'moral worlds.'"[26] Given this variability, even if one wants to assert a normative claim that moral agents ought to act according to universal, objective moral rules, the descriptive claim that in fact humans deliberate about and account for morals using such frameworks is dubious.

Of course, arguing that this extreme heterogeneity has metaethical implications is not to commit the naturalistic fallacy; the fact that morality seems to vary across cultures and contexts does not in and of itself imply that moral agents ought not act according to "universal" principles and rules of morality. But if the existence of such principles and rules is dubious, it is fair to criticize an ethical theory that indisputably relies on the notion that a universal, common morality or set of principles both exists and is knowable. If such principles or general rules are either not knowable or not understandable across different moral worlds, moral agents can hardly be charged with the obligation to be guided by them. As Mackie puts it, "the argument from relativity has some force simply because the actual variations in the moral codes are more readily explained by the hypothesis that they reflect ways of life than by the hypothesis that they express perceptions, most of them seriously inadequate and badly distorted, of objective values."[27]

A more devastating critique of principlism, which Turner also adopts, is the notion that principlism in morals is unhelpful as an action guide.[28] My own difficulty with moral principlism is that, in my view, it is either false or it is thin. Either reference to a common stock of principles is dubious for the reasons Turner suggests, or reliance on a notion of "autonomy" or "justice" requires for its commonality a level of abstraction that renders it of little use in guiding action in concrete, particular circumstances. A basic implication of phenomenology is that our experiences are irreducibly local and particular; our social worlds are inevitably shaped by the particular relationships, contexts, and networks in which we are embedded. Thus, giving content to the acts required or prohibited by a commitment to justice depends greatly on the local, particular social and moral worlds that we inhabit. Accordingly, even if moral agents from divergent moral worlds might share a broad commitment to "justice," they might well understand what "justice" requires in any given situation entirely differently. Thus, the appeal to a common or shared sense of justice is thin, because it is only in context and in practice that thick notions of justice can be conceptualized. As Turner puts it:

> Even if some highly abstract notion of the four principles could be found in a core common morality, this shared understanding at the level of abstract principles need not in any way promote agreement during the process of specifying and balancing principles. For example, although it is possible to respect "autonomy" in general or to defend "justice" in the abstract, it is quite another matter to defend specific autonomous choices that are understood to lead to particular practical outcomes.[29]

This has deep relevance for the inevitably local, particularized problems that tend to dominate the attention of bioethicists and bioethics practice because "[d]ifferent kinds of disputes occur in encounters within clinical settings."[30] Reliance on a general stock of principles, or a common morality

> contains little practical advice concerning how to navigate situations in which there is substantial disagreement about initial presumptions and 'reasonable' conclusions at the level of policy and practice. This is a rather significant shortcoming given that the United States contains many religious traditions, ethnic groups, and cultures where there can be different substantive accounts of moral practices and policies.[31]

As such, "social theorists who emphasize the local, temporal character of 'moral worlds' challenge accounts presuming the existence of a universal moral Esperanto."[32] Moreover, both the practical problems that attend principlism in bioethics and its difficulty in accounting for the undeniable fact of cultural relativism imply problems of ethical imperialism, a charge that has long been leveled at dominant (principlist) traditions of Western bioethics.[33] For example, Turner observes that Beauchamp and Childress—who are hardly alone in this respect—

> mention human rights as examples of cross-cultural moral norms that fall within boundaries of the common morality. However, the language

of human rights is not a transhistorical, transcultural phenomena found in all communities throughout time. . . . Indeed, some critics of the rhetoric of human rights argue that conceptions of human rights emphasizing individualism constitute a form of "Western imperialism" that fails to acknowledge sufficiently communitarian understandings of duties and obligations.[34]

Ultimately, whatever its flaws in helping stakeholders find meaning in experiences of health and illness in general, principlism is especially poorly suited to illuminating lived experiences of pain because, as conceptualized in the dominant traditions of bioethics, it has difficulty incorporating and/ or accommodating local, particular, specific circumstances. By virtue of the generality of principlism and related moral traditions, focus is directed away from the local social worlds that characterize the phenomenology of pain. This is in part why the phenomenology of pain is so crucial to formulating an ethical framework for pain policy; in such an account, the embodied person in pain is by definition central.

THE ETHICAL IMPLICATIONS OF THE PHENOMENOLOGY OF PAIN

How is understanding the phenomenon of pain helpful in producing ethical policy and practice as to pain?

Recall that for many pain sufferers, their lived experiences are marked by isolation, stigma, and exile, even from their own bodies. Thus, in phenomenologic terms, the primary means of alleviating the pain patient's existential suffering is to bring them back into the social world and into a sense of community. If part of what is so devastating about pain is its language-destroying, isolating nature, repatriating pain sufferers from their exile might be an important component of healing the pain sufferer.[35] Even the very act of listening to the pain sufferer and taking a narrative can be an important step in bringing the pain sufferer into society: "An epistemic bridge is built. In this restoration of intersubjective understanding, the relief of pain has already begun."[36]

Two other examples may help to illuminate the ethical significance of building the epistemic bridge to which Leder refers. First, there is the healing tradition of the laying on of hands, which has both diverse and ancient roots.[37] Wuthnow notes that "[c]ave paintings in the Pyrenees 15,000 years old depict such healing as do written records of 5,000 years ago."[38] In the medieval and early modern Western incarnations of this ritual, the illness sufferer, who characteristically lived with disfiguring illnesses like scrofula, sought out the king's healing touch, generally referred to as 'royal touch.'[39] Multiple French and English kings utilized royal touch during the Late Middle Ages.[40] But why seek out the king? Why not the physician or professional healer? Why not the clergy? What was it about the king's touch that was deemed to heal?

The superficial answer is that in much of Europe during the Middle Ages, kingship was allied with divinity, such that supplicating before the king was, in an important sense, seeking divine intervention in one's suffering.[41] The deeper answer, more relevant to my purpose here, is that the medieval and early modern monarch was broadly identified as the body politic, as the society and community itself. Therefore, in a phenomenological and ritualistic sense, for the king to lay hands on the disfigured, isolated illness sufferer meant that the sufferer had literally been brought back into the body politic, and hence into society. The sufferer had therefore been healed in a profoundly phenomenologic sense. It is a minimalist conception indeed that dismisses the power of this form of healing because of its apparent lack of clinical efficacy.[42] Indeed, part of my point is that, as important as clinical efficacy is—and I do not mean for a moment to discount its importance—there are dimensions of illness and pain for which a narrow focus on clinical interventions and efficacy cannot account.

This basic idea recurs in the growing literature on the phenomenology of illness and its ethical implications. Murray argues that emphasis on the lived experiences of illness can help "reorient ethics towards the body in crisis, toward the address of a body that speaks."[43] Doing so promises the possibility of breaking "free from the ossified language of institutional bioethics, with its relatively static principles, to invent a language for ethics that makes sense of lived bodies."[44]

It is important to note that the repatriation from the exile imposed by pain that many phenomenologically minded commentators recommend has ethical content. To understand the isolation imposed by pain and to actively seek to restore the sufferer into a compassionate community is to act virtuously, to practice excellence in healing. vanHooft reasons that

> in the case of pain, the ethical challenge is to reopen the patient's world so as to break open the isolation into which their pain has forced them. . . . The pain of the other, which tends to their self-enclosure, must be made into an opening through which the care of the clinician flows through to the patient.[45]

This reopening, of course, must be undertaken with great sensitivity and caution, for the pain sufferer is frequently isolated, vulnerable, and wary. "The clinician must bring to this encounter a mode of apprehension which does not objectify the other or their pain."[46] Yet the ethical significance of such a reopening can only be understood through a phenomenology of pain, through apprehension of the ways in which pain shapes the pain sufferer's lifeworld.

Although repatriation through listening may seem easy enough for the provider, this is a dangerous assumption.[47] Too many providers simply do not *hear* their patients' pain talk. I have already documented the existence of a profound communication gap between pain sufferers and their physicians.[48] Akin to Heath's analysis of the preeminence of diagnosis in communication about pain between patients and physicians, Thomas and Johnson note that for many physicians 'listening' "mean[s] hearing words as diagnostic cues, not placing the words into the context of the patient's life world."[49] Leder explains that "[t]he contemporary medical care system does not always foster this restoration of the world. A callous or uncommunicative doctor can heighten rather than relieve the patient's sense of isolation."[50] Moreover, one should not doubt the importance of diagnosis; Charles Rosenberg suggests that it is the very linchpin of the process that knits together the chief players, institutions, and strategies for defining, categorizing, and assimilating experiences of disease itself in the U.S.[51]

In an important sense, the moral objectivism that dominates principlism and common morality bioethics mirrors the emphasis on objectivity that dominates contemporary understandings of pain. This is not altogether surprising when one considers the attempts to naturalize moral philosophy in general and bioethics in particular. Without passing judgment on the merits of such projects writ large, the smaller claim issued here is that such objectivism is poorly suited to accounting for the body in pain and the ethical issues that attend the general failures in the response to that phenomenon in the U.S. Havi Carel notes that a phenomenological approach to illness is important precisely because it counters the "naturalistic foundations of medicine" that have been a primary subject in this book.[52] One could argue that such an approach is at least an important counterpart, if not a counter, to some of the objectivizing, principlist traditions in bioethical analyses of pain.

The second example of the ethical significance of the phenomenology of pain is a contemporary version of the royal laying on of hands: touch therapy. Through touch therapy, the phenomenological use of "laying on hands" to bring illness sufferers back into the body politic continues to the present: "Therapeutic touch is a healing modality practiced by thousands of registered nurses."[53] Long derided as another unproven complementary and alternative treatment, the tone has changed as the evidence base increased. There is now solid evidence that different forms of touching— massage, cradling, etc.—can be clinically beneficial in a variety of illness encounters. Cochrane reviews indicate reasonable evidence of benefit for the use of touch therapy in treating pain,[54] dementia,[55] and chronic/recurrent headache.[56] Moreover, systematic reviews also suggest some benefit to infants under six months of age from skin-to-skin contact with their mothers.[57] Finally, there is a great deal of evidence outside that produced by randomized controlled trials[58] suggesting benefit in a wide array of illness scenarios.[59] Although there is no shortage of clinical and molecular explanations for these findings, given the insights of the phenomenology of illness and pain, it should be fairly obvious, and yet obvious in important ways, why the act of touching another human being can be therapeutic.

The criticisms of principlism and common morality bioethics noted in this chapter often argue that such approaches are ill-suited to account for the variety of attitudes, beliefs, and practices across local, particular worlds. Pain presents an excellent example of a defining illness experience that varies in just such ways. Thus Giordano, Engebretson, and Benedikter argue that

> any practical consideration of an ethics of pain medicine must also recognize (1) the effects of culture on the event, phenomenon, and experience of pain; (2) the distinctions that are evoked by the culture of medicine (vs. the culture of patienthood); and (3) how geographic, social, and temporal variances affect these cultural dynamics.[60]

Accordingly, any attempts to improve the undertreatment of pain in the U.S. that do not account for the social and cultural meanings of pain in American society are unlikely to succeed. The second point underscores another key aspect of my argument: that providers as well as pain sufferers (and caregivers) participate in framing a culture of pain in which pain is undertreated. Note that this is *not* to imply that pain sufferers are responsible for such undertreatment, but simply that the larger social and cultural narratives I have traced here shape the meaning of pain for providers, pain sufferers, and caregivers alike.[61]

While the role these larger conceptions of objectivity, illness, and the power of the visible play in American and biomedical culture are crucial to understanding the meaning of pain in society, at the same time, it is the local worlds that actors move through that frame ethical significance. This meshes with Giordano, Engrebetson, and Benedikter's point number three above, that a myriad of *local* variances— "geographic, social, and temporal"—shapes and informs the meaning persons attach to pain in different ways. Thus the meaning of pain, like many intricate, complicated phenomena is shaped both by larger social trajectories and by the particular features of the sufferer's local moral and social world. In addition, as I have noted, Leder suggests that if health care providers were more attuned to the particular, subjective pain experiences their patients reported, not only would pain be likely to be treated better, but the provider would be more likely to *heal* the patient, as opposed to merely treat the disease.[62]

Finally, it is of course true that the objective modalities that characterize Western and American science and medicine have had powerful salutary effects. Inasmuch as these modalities can improve the treatment of pain and reduce unnecessary human suffering, their use should be encouraged. But a central aim of my project is to suggest what such a turn has diminished, what other ways of knowing and thinking and conceptualizing pain and illness have been lost or reduced in the process.[63] Thus, while it would be absurd to deny the utility of objectification in the treatment of pain, it does not follow that the optimal means of healing the pain sufferer is by objectifying modalities and interventions. Moreover, some methods of objectification, such as many kinds of diagnostic imaging techniques, may turn out to be of little use in treating certain kinds of pain, and may instead do much to decenter, stigmatize, and ultimately augment the person-in-pain's suffering.[64]

CONCLUSION

The phenomenology of pain embodies the primary objective of this project, which is to center an analysis of why pain is so dramatically undertreated in the U.S. on the pain sufferer. This is neither trivial nor facile; the clinical gaze inexorably directs focus away from the subject in pain and towards attempts to diagnose, to view the objects that are presumed to cause the experience of pain. Moreover, the dominant approach to ethics and pain policy in the United States focuses almost entirely on the opioid regulatory regime, which centers the physician-prescriber. Phenomenology is important to the ethics of pain because it implies that the primary locus of ethical significance is the being-in-the-world, the particular subject moving through their local, social world and experiencing and understanding the meaning of their pain in terms of these local worlds. Principlism, objectivism, and generalism in morals almost by definition are poorly suited to accounting for these contextual factors, although again, this is not to suggest such approaches could not be used in developing a richer account. However, the specific modes and practices of such ethical approaches in bioethics do not, in my view, inspire confidence that such an enriched framework is forthcoming.

What I have tried to do in this project is to suggest the primacy of some of the social and cultural factors that animate the meaning of pain in American society, and to explain how the dominance of objectivity in American society and in the culture of biomedicine is a major reason why pain continues to be undertreated. With such an understanding, what remains to be done is to translate this evidence into policy recommendations that justify a hope that improvement in treating pain in the United States is possible. This task is the subject of the final two chapters in my analysis.

NOTES

1. John Leslie Mackie, "The Subjectivity of Values," in *Morality and the Good Life*, ed. Thomas L. Carson and Paul K. Moser (New York, NY: Oxford University Press, 1997), 299.
2. For example, O'Neill agrees with many critics that much of the discourse within bioethics regarding autonomy is deficient, and more so, that it is not in keeping with a deep understanding of Kantian moral theory. Onora O'Neill, *Autonomy and Trust in Bioethics* (Cambridge, UK: Cambridge University Press, 2002).
3. Tom L. Beauchamp, and James R. Childress, *Principles of Biomedical Ethics*, 6th ed. (New York, NY: Oxford University Press, 2008).
4. Documenting this dominance has been a primary objective of what Raymond DeVries terms the sociology of bioethics. Raymond DeVries, "How Can We

Help? From 'Sociology in' to 'Sociology of' Bioethics," *Journal of Law, Medicine & Ethics* 32, no. 2 (2004): 279–92; Raymond DeVries, "Toward a Sociology of Bioethics," *Qualitative Sociology* 18, no. 1 (1995): 119–28.

5. Oonagh Corrigan, "Empty Ethics: The Problem with Informed Consent," *Sociology of Health & Illness* 25, no. 7 (2003): 768–92.

6. John H. Evans, "A Sociological Account of the Growth of Principlism," *Hastings Center Report* 30, no. 5 (2000): 36.

7. Ibid.

8. Ibid.

9. Ibid.

10. Ibid.

11. Ibid.

12. Leigh Turner, "Zones of Consensus and Zones of Conflict: Questioning the 'Common Morality' Presumption in Bioethics," *Kennedy Institute of Ethics Journal* 13, no. 3 (2003): 193–218.

13. Dancy, *Ethics Without Principles*, 7.

14. Mackie, "The Subjectivity of Values," 299.

15. Ibid., 301.

16. Justin Felux, "A Defense of Moral Objectivism," *Symposia: The Online Philosophy Journal,* accessed June 5, 2012, from http://journal.ilovephilosophy.com/Article/A-Defense-of-Moral-Objectivism/10.

17. Ibid.

18. Ibid. However, Mitchell Silver's conception of moral objectivism expressly rejects the criteria of subject-independence. It is nevertheless principlistic: "Moral objectivism … is the view that a single set of principles determines the permissibility of any action, and the correctness of any judgment regarding an action's permissibility." Mitchell Silver, "Our Morality: A Defense of Moral Objectivism," *Philosophy Now: A Magazine of Ideas,* accessed July 23, 2012, from http://philosophynow.org/issues/83/Our_Morality_A_Defense_of_Moral_Objectivism.

19. Ibid.

20. Mackie, "The Subjectivity of Values," 291.

21. Ibid., 292.

22. Mark Johnson, *The Moral Imagination: Implications of Cognitive Science for Ethics* (Chicago, IL: University of Chicago Press, 1993), 17.

23. Ibid., 30.

24. Turner, "Zones of Consensus," 196.

25. Ibid., 197 (citations omitted).

26. Ibid., 206.

27. Mackie, "The Subjectivity of Values," 302.

28. For a succinct recent exposition of this argument that builds on Turner's arguments from moral pluralism, see Marvin H. Lee, "The Problem of 'Thick in Status, Thin in Content' in Beauchamp and Childress' Principlism," *Journal of Medical Ethics* 36, no. 9 (2010): 525–8.

29. Turner, "Zones of Consensus," 207.

30. Ibid., 208.

31. Ibid.

32. Ibid., 206.

33. E.g., Heather Widdows, "Is Global Ethics Moral Neo-Colonialism? An Investigation of the Issue in the Context of Bioethics," *Bioethics* 21, no. 6 (July 2007): 305–15; Paul Farmer and Nicole Gastineau Campos, "New Malaise: Bioethics and Human Rights in the Global Era," *American Journal of Law, Medicine & Ethics* 32, no. 2 (Summer 2004): 243–51; Erich H. Loewy, "Bioethics: Past, Present, and an Open Future," *Cambridge Quarterly of Health Care Ethics* 11, no. 4 (Fall 2002): 388–97; Solomon R. Benatar, "Reflections

and Recommendations on Research Ethics in Developing Countries," *Social Science & Medicine* 54, no. 7 (April 2002): 1131–41; and Paquitade Zulueta, "Randomised Placebo-controlled trials and HIV-infected Pregnant Women in Developing Countries: Ethical Imperialism or Unethical Exploitation," *Bioethics* 15, no. 4 (August 2001): 289–311.

34. Turner, "Zones of Consensus," 207.
35. Goldberg, "Exilic Effects of Illness and Pain."
36. Leder, "The Experience of Pain and Its Clinical Implications"; see also Rita Charon, "A Narrative Medicine for Pain," in *Narrative, Pain, and Suffering,* eds. Daniel B. Carr, John David Loeser, and David B. Morris (Seattle, WA: IASP Press, 2003), 29–44.
37. Elizabeth L. Lewton and Victoria Bydone, "Identity and Healing in Three Navajo Religious Traditions: Sa'ah Naagháí Bik'eh Hózh," *Medical Anthropology Quarterly* 14, no. 4 (December 2000): 476–97; Sara Wuthnow, "Healing Touch Controversies," *Journal of Religion and Health* 36, no. 3 (September 1997): 221–30; and John G. Bruhn, "The Doctor's Touch: Tactile Communication in the Doctor-Patient Relationship," *Southern Medical Journal* 71, no. 12 (December 1978): 1469–73.
38. Wuthnow, "Healing Touch Controversies," 221–2 (citation omitted).
39. The phenomenon of royal touch is exhaustively analyzed by the great medievalist Marc Bloch in *The Royal Touch: Monarchy and Miracles in France and England,* trans. James E. Anderson (New York, NY: Dorset Press, 1990).
40. Ibid.
41. This obviously encroached upon ecclesiastical prerogative. Ibid.; Wuthnow, "Healing Touch Controversies."
42. On the fallacy of conflating clinical efficacy with social and cultural efficacy, see Rosenberg, "The Therapeutic Revolution." In my view, this essay on the therapeutic revolution of the nineteenth century is one of the most important works in the history of medicine and the medical humanities of the last 35 years.
43. Stuart J. Murray, "Phenomenology, Ethics, and the Crisis of the Lived Body," *Nursing Philosophy* 13 (2012): 289–94, 292.
44. Ibid.
45. vanHooft, "Pain and Communication," 260.
46. Ibid.
47. Goldberg, "Job and the Stigmatization of Chronic Pain"; Goldberg, "Exilic Effects of Illness and Pain."
48. E.g., Jackson, "Stigma, Liminality, and Chronic Pain"; Thomas and Johnson, "A Phenomenologic Study of Chronic Pain"; Baszanger, *Inventing Pain Medicine;* and Heath, "Pain Talk," 115–16.
49. Thomas and Johnson, "A Phenomenologic Study of Chronic Pain," 695.
50. Leder, "The Experience of Pain," 101.
51. Charles E. Rosenberg, "The Tyranny of Diagnosis: Specific Entities and Individual Experience," *The Milbank Quarterly* 80, no. 2 (June 2002): 237–60.
52. Havi Carel, "Phenomenology and its Application in Medicine," *Theoretical Medicine and Bioethics* 32 (2011): 33–46, 41–2.
53. Wuthnow, "Healing Touch Controversies," 226.
54. Pui Shan So, Yu Jiang, and Ying Qin, "Touch Therapies for Pain Relief in Adults," *Cochrane Database of Systematic Reviews* 4, Art. No.: CD006535 (October 2008), doi:10.1002/14651858.CD006535.pub2, accessed June 1, 2012, from http://dx.doi.org/10.1002/14651858.CD006535.pub2; Andrea D. Furlan, Marta Imamura, Trish Dryden, and Emma Irvin, "Massage for Low-Back Pain," *Cochrane Database of Systematic Reviews* 6, Art. No.: CD001929 (May 2010), accessed June 1, 2012, from http://dx.doi.org/10.1002/14651858.CD001929.pub2.

55. Niels Viggo Hansen, Torben Jørgensen, and Lisbeth Ørtenblad, "Massage and Touch for Dementia," *Cochrane Database of Systematic Reviews* 4, Art. No.: CD004989 (May 2008), doi:10.1002/14651858.CD004989.pub2, accessed June 1, 2012, from http://dx.doi.org/10.1002/14651858.CD004989.pub2.

56. Gert Brønfort, Niels Nilsson, Mitchell Haas, Roni L. Evans, Charles H. Goldsmith, Willem J. J. Assendelft, and Lex M. Bouter, "Non-invasive Physical Treatments for Chronic/Recurrent Headache," *Cochrane Database of Systematic Reviews* 3, Art. No.: CD001878 (August 2008), doi:10.1002/14651858.CD001878.pub2, accessed June 1, 2012, from http://dx.doi.org/10.1002/14651858.CD001878.pub2.

57. Elizabeth R. Moore, Gene C Anderson, Nils Bergman, and Therese Dowswell, "Early Skin-to-Skin Contact for Mothers and Their Healthy Newborn Infants," *Cochrane Database of Systematic Reviews* 3, Art. No.: CD003519 (March 2012), doi:10.1002/14651858.CD003519.pub2, accessed June 1, 2012, from http://dx.doi.org/10.1002/14651858.CD003519.pub2; and Angela Underdown, Jane Barlow, Vincent Chung, and Sarah Stewart-Brown, "Massage Intervention for Promoting Mental and Physical Health in Infants Aged Under Six Months," *Cochrane Database of Systematic Reviews* 4, Art. No.: CD005038 (November 2008), doi:10.1002/14651858.CD005038.pub2, last accessed June 1, 2012, from http://dx.doi.org/10.1002/14651858.CD005038.pub2.

58. On the problems with assuming that only evidence produced via RCTs "counts" in healing, see e.g., Grossman, "A Couple of the Nasties Lurking in Evidence-Based Medicine"; Adam La Caze, "Evidence-Based Medicine Can't Be . . ."; Brody, Miller, and Bogdan-Lovis, "Evidence-Based Medicine: Watching out for Its Friends"; and Upshur, "Looking for Rules in a World of Exceptions." In addition, vol. 22, no. 4 of *Social Epistemology* (Oct.–Dec. 2008) is a theme issue addressing evidence-based medicine. Jason Grossman lists as "Dumb Claim Number 1" the idea that "[a]nyrandomised controlled trial (RCT) gives us better evidence than any other study." Grossman, "A Couple of the Nasties Lurking in Evidence-Based Medicine," 335.

59. Lesley Cullen and Julie Barlow, "'Kiss, Cuddle, Squeeze': The Experiences and Meaning of Touch among Parents of Children with Autism Attending a Touch Therapy Programme," *Journal of Child Health Care* 6, no. 3 (September 2002): 171–81; Tiffany Field, *Touch Therapy* (London, UK: Churchill Livingstone, 2000); Paulette Sansone and Louise Schmitt, "Providing Tender Touch Massage to Elderly Nursing Home Residents: A Demonstration Project," *Geriatric Nursing* 21, no. 6 (November 2000): 303–8; and Maria Hernandez-Reif, Tiffany Field, Josh Krasnegor, Elena Martinez, Morton Schwartzman, and Kunjana Mavunda, "Children with Cystic Fibrosis Benefit from Massage Therapy," *Journal of Pediatric Psychology* 24, no. 2 (April/May 1999): 175–81.

60. James Giordano, Joan C. Engebretson, and Roland Benedikter, "Culture, Subjectivity, and the Ethics of Patient-Centered Pain Care," *Cambridge Quarterly of Health Care Ethics* 18, no. 1 (January 2009): 48.

61. I discuss this issue in detail in Chapter 8 (this volume).

62. Leder, "The Experience of Pain."

63. E.g., Arthur Kleinman, "Opening Remarks: Pain as Experience," in *Pain and Its Transformations: The Interface of Biology and Culture*, eds. Sarah Coakley and Kay Kaufman Shelemay (Cambridge, MA: Harvard University Press, 2007), 17–20; Kleinman, "Pain as Resistance"; and Hamlin, "Predisposing Causes."

64. This argument is taken up in earnest in Chapter 8 (this volume).

Section IV

Towards Ethical, Evidence-Based Pain Policy

In the Introduction, I argued that the Renaissance humanists were early translational researchers. The term "translation" is something of a catch-phrase in academic medicine and science these days, emphasizing the need to translate the knowledge produced via scientific and clinical research into practices that will benefit individuals and communities.[1]

The translational question lies at the heart of this project. The undertreatment of pain in the U.S. is not a function of insufficient technical knowledge and capacity. If so, it follows that the problem is at its root one of translation. This is one reason why a health humanities approach is particularly well-suited to analysis of the problem. However, mere analysis of the problem is inconsistent with the ethos of practical engagement embodied by the humanists. As worthwhile as it might be to identify some of the primary social and cultural factors in the undertreatment of pain, a health humanities approach demands more. The evidence must be translated into a way that practically engages the nonacademic world. There are many media for doing so; the one I utilize in this final section is public health policy. Why choose policy? Policy by definition affects a multiplicity of communities and persons, and has the potential to change behavior across and within various sectors. For such reasons, policy development is widely regarded as a core function of public health in the U.S.[2] Under the best of circumstances, policy can have a broad impact on shaping a society's collective answer to Aristotle's foundational question, "how shall we live?"

In this chapter and the one that follows, I bring together the various strands of analysis and disciplinary tools I have been working with into a bundle of public health policies that incorporate in their structure key ideas related to the meaning of pain in the U.S. However well-intentioned, currently, dominant policy approaches leave out such an assessment, and as such, are not tailored to the root social and cultural causes that drive the undertreatment of pain. While I have mentioned this problem throughout my analysis, this chapter is devoted to a focused assessment of some of the dominant approaches to ethical pain policy. In highlighting the strengths and weaknesses of these policies, I will contextualize my own pain policy recommendations, which follow in Chapter 8 (this volume).

7   Opioids and Pain Policy

INTRODUCTION

In this chapter, I lay out and criticize what I perceive as the dominant policy approach to pain, which centers on the opioid regulatory scheme. My criticisms do not necessarily arise from a fundamental disagreement with the objectives of this approach, but rather from the evidence that it has had little measurable impact on the undertreatment of pain in the U.S. I then provide a brief analysis, picking up on themes and arguments advanced in the first five chapters, of why the dominant policy approach is deficient.

In thinking about pain and its treatment, we see at least two major public health problems: prescription drug misuse and the undertreatment of pain. While this book has focused largely on the latter, there is no doubt that the former is an enormous problem, and the statistics are in their own way almost as staggering as those regarding the inequitable undertreatment of pain. According to the Center for Disease Control (CDC), drug overdose fatalities have increased annually for the last 11 consecutive years, from 16,849 deaths in 1999 to 38,329 in 2010. Sixty percent of these deaths involved pharmaceutical drugs, with 75 percent of pharmaceutical-related deaths resulting from opioids.

Yet my principal argument in this chapter, and indeed, in this book, is that these are in fact distinct public health problems. In the U.S., well-intentioned stakeholders have proceeded to conflate the problems, apparently believing that if we resolve our difficulties in managing the safe and effective utilization of opioid analgesics, we will substantially resolve our problems in treating pain. This is error. Both of these issues are serious public health problems, but they are not the same problem. We will not resolve the undertreatment of pain in the U.S. by striking the right balance in the management of opioid analgesics, regardless of whether that balance tilts in favor of liberalization or restriction of their availability. This chapter is devoted to explaining why this is so, and hence why I eschew an approach that focuses on opioids. Attention to both problems is certainly justified, but in this book, I am squarely focused on the undertreatment of pain.

At the outset, it is useful to lay out the state-of-the-art regarding the safety and efficacy of opioids for the treatment of pain. As there is reasonable evidence that long-term usage opioids for pain may be only marginally effective for a general population of pain sufferers, this undermines further the notion that liberalizing access to opioids will dramatically improve the undertreatment of pain.

Finally, I end the chapter by surveying some of the issues related to the meaning of opioids in American society. This general lack of an assessment of the meaning of opioids is an additional deficiency in the dominant policy approach. Even if I am mistaken and the opioid regulatory regime is critical to improving the treatment of pain, attempts to reshape and correct the policy scheme are unlikely to have significant impact if they are divorced from a deep understanding of the meaning of opioids. Although I do not provide such an analysis here because I ultimately remain unconvinced that such an approach is central to improving the undertreatment of pain in the U.S., I nevertheless close the chapter by sketching some features of what such an account might look like. This last segment of the chapter addresses some of the furor over the prosecution of opioid prescribers, which far and away generates the lion's share of the focus on the undertreatment of pain in the U.S. Such focus is unjustified, not because it is irrelevant to the culture of pain, but rather because it is unlikely to improve the undertreatment of pain in the U.S.

THE DOMINANT POLICY APPROACH TO PAIN: BALANCE IN OPIOID REGULATIONS

There is exactly one entity in the U.S. specifically devoted to pain policy that is expressly housed at an academic medical center: the Pain & Policy Studies Group (PPSG), affiliated with the University of Wisconsin Paul B. Carbone Cancer Center. For over 20 years, the PPSG has dominated academic and political discussions of pain policy in the U.S.

Since 1997, the PPSG has produced several editions of two documents whose influence on pain policy can barely be overstated. These documents are the "Achieving Balance" reports, which include a "Progress Report Card" and an "Evaluation Guide" containing profiles of each U.S. state and the federal government. The criteria for evaluation center on the government entity's compliance with the guiding principle of the PPSG, which is "balance" in regulation of opioid analgesics.[3] "Balance" is sought between the legitimate law enforcement aim of preventing the abuse and diversion of powerful narcotics like opioids, and the key role opioid analgesics play in the effective treatment of pain.[4] As stated in the Introduction (this volume), it is perfectly appropriate to seek balance in public health policy of any kind, and the PPSG documents are valuable tools in this endeavor.

However, there are significant limitations to the PPSG approach. The first major problem is the unstated assumption that achieving balance in opioid policy is the primary means of improving the undertreatment of pain in the U.S. The reason this assumption is problematic is because a focus on opioid policy leaves opaque the role that social and cultural beliefs, attitudes, and practices regarding the meaning of pain play in its undertreatment. The example I provided in the Introduction (this volume) noted the tendency of elderly persons in the U.S. to underreport their pain, which is a significant barrier to effective treatment.[5] There is little reason to believe that achieving balance in the opioid regulatory scheme will remedy this problem.

Second, a focus on opioid policy inevitably centers on the opioid prescriber, which in the U.S., is exclusively the physician. This is a serious problem because common attitudes, practices, and beliefs about the meaning of pain are part of a cultural frame shared by pain sufferers, caregivers, and nonphysician health care providers (of which elderly populations tending to underreport their pain is an excellent example). Focus simply on the prescribers obscures the larger contexts that deeply influence practices and beliefs towards pain and its treatment. Thus, for example, pain sufferers frequently join physicians in the attempt to objectify their own pain, self-stigmatize, and doubt the pain talk of fellow pain sufferers.

Third, the efforts to achieve balance in the opioid regulatory scheme typically do not explain or account for the reasons why opioid policy has historically been and remains unbalanced in the U.S.[6] That is, to reconfigure opioid policies in ways that come closer to an ideal state of balance, it seems important to tailor these efforts to address the root causes that have driven the imbalance in opioid policy. Policy that is not so tailored is unlikely to have the practical effect intended or hoped for, and is in my view a central reason why the best efforts of the PPSG and its allies do not seem to have had the expected and hoped-for impact as of the current date. C. Stratton Hill, Jr., a retired cancer physician and pain specialist who has been advocating for improved pain treatment for over three decades, maintains that an approach that focuses almost exclusively on tweaking the regulatory scheme is simply doing what was tried over 30 years ago, with little success.[7]

Why does the PPSG's approach to pain policy focuses almost exclusively on the opioid regulatory regime? On one level, the answer is obvious: for centuries if not millennia, opioids have been a frontline therapy for the effective treatment of many kinds of pain. Yet other factors likely contribute, and do so in important ways. For example, Richard deGrandpre coined the phrase "behavioral pharmacologism" to refer to the American tendency to see health problems primarily if not exclusively in context of pharmaceuticals.[8] That this behavior is encouraged by the pharmaceutical industry is also beyond dispute. In context of pain, this operates to shape policy discourse at the highest levels, such that even well-intentioned groups like the PPSG tend to see the problem of and potential solutions to the undertreatment of pain primarily in terms of the availability of pharmaceutical drugs.[9]

There is little question that opioids remain relevant for treating pain today, but an increasing body of evidence suggests that the efficacy of opioid analgesics for different kinds of pain is uncertain at best. If this evidence is legitimate, it obviously suggests a fourth reason for contending that an undue policy focus on opioid regulation is unlikely to substantially improve the undertreatment of pain: opioids themselves, however important, are not even the *clinical* answer to the undertreatment of pain. Examining this evidence briefly is important to thinking about the strengths and weaknesses of the "balance" approach.

EVIDENCE RELATED TO THE USE
OF OPIOIDS IN TREATING PAIN

The present state of the art regarding the use of opioids for treating pain is in flux. There is little question both that opioids remain an important therapy and that the total volume of opioid dispensation has increased dramatically over the last two decades. Such an increase has coincided with a dramatic increase in the total number of fatalities attributed to prescription drugs, and although there are likely myriad reasons for the latter, it strains credulity to deny any causal connection between the liberalization of the opioid regime and the significant increase in deaths and other adverse drug events. Given the significant public health risks, there is reason for demanding significant evidence of clinical benefit for the utilization of such opioids.

> Yet Deshpande et al. observe that despite the fact that the use of opioids . . . remain[s] a controversial issue in the management of chronic non-cancer pain, and chronic [low-back pain] in particular, there is a steadily growing trend toward prescribing opioids for the management of [chronic non-cancer pain]. Market data indicate that since 2000, long- and short-acting opioids experienced a 26.5 percent and 39 percent compounded annual growth rate, respectively.[10]

The controversy over the extent of the efficacy of opioids for chronic non-malignant pain seems to have grown concomitant to its usage.[11] In their systematic review of the efficacy of opioids in improving pain or function in persons with chronic low-back pain, Deshpande et al. conclude that "there was no statistically significant difference between [subjects given strong opioids like oxycodone and morphine and subjects given naproxen] for either pain relief or functional improvement."[12]

Similarly, Noble et al. note that while many pain sufferers discontinue long-term usage of opioids for chronic nonmalignant pain due to either or both adverse effects and/or insufficient pain relief, only weak evidence exists to support such long-term usage.[13] Moreover, both Deshpande et al. and Noble et al. note the paucity of high-quality studies that would generate confidence in assessments of the safety and efficacy of long-term usage of opioids for chronic nonmalignant pain. Ultimately, Deshpande et al. suggest that "[a]s the pendulum swings from an 'opiophobic' to an 'opiophilic' society, physicians should question whether the current trend is based on evidence or simply the outcries of well-intentioned patient advocates and aggressive marketing efforts by the pharmaceutical industry."[14]

Here, two points are relevant. First, it is becoming increasingly less plausible, if ever it was so, to suggest that opioids are a panacea for virtually any kind of chronic pain. Given the multivalence of pain,[15] it is unsurprising that no single intervention suffices to ameliorate all or even most different kinds of pain. This suggests even further reason for doubting that undue focus on the opioid regulatory regime is likely to result in substantial improvement in the undertreatment of pain in the U.S. If in fact opioids are more limited in relieving (especially chronic) pain than we might have imagined, it follows that even a perfectly balanced opioid regulatory scheme may not result in significantly better treatment of American pain sufferers.

The second point arising from this more complicated picture of the efficacy of opioids is whether such a view undermines the claim I have advanced throughout this project, that we generally enjoy the technical capacity to treat pain far better than we currently do. One could argue that if opioids are less effective than had previously been imagined in treating chronic pain, perhaps the ability to ameliorate pain is correspondingly lesser as well.

This argument seems plausible, but breaks down upon closer examination. The notion that because opioids are not a cure-all for pain we lack the technical ability to ameliorate pain far better than is currently done is question-begging inasmuch as it implies that our capacity to relieve pain is mostly a function of facility with opioids. The briefest glance at any textbook or manual on clinical pain management is sufficient to disprove this idea, as it is almost universally acknowledged that effective treatment of pain requires multimodal, multidisciplinary efforts.[16] Despite the apparent emphasis on the use of opioids in the treatment of pain, there is no serious clinical suggestion that the exclusive use of opioids is an effective means of treating pain. Numerous other interventions, pharmacologic and nonpharmacologic, are of demonstrated efficacy in treating certain kinds of pain. Acetaminophen, aspirin, and nonsteroidal anti-inflammatory drugs are all effective analgesics for some kinds of pain, as are massage,[17] yoga,[18] and cognitive behavioral therapy (especially with regard to improving mood in chronic pain sufferers).[19] The idea that we enjoy the technical capacity in the U.S. to treat pain far better than we do is based on the variety of approaches and interventions that demonstrate safety and efficacy in treating pain. Opioids are one of the most important of these interventions, but they are nevertheless simply one tool in the multimodal, multidisciplinary pain treatment toolbox. Given the scope of these tools, there is no technical reason why, for example, 40–80 percent of residents in long-term care facilities should suffer daily, persistent pain.[20]

Thus far in this chapter, I have suggested some reasons for doubting that a single-minded focus on opioid regulation is likely to substantially improve the undertreatment of pain in the U.S. However, even if I am wrong, and pursuing balance in the opioid regulatory scheme is the most effective means of improving the undertreatment of pain, it is still crucial to understand that regulatory regime as the result of a constant, dynamic interaction of various actors and stakeholders regarding the distribution of powerful narcotics. Understanding something about the meaning of opioids in American society is therefore integral in pursuing a policy agenda regarding those opioids. Fortunately, there is no shortage of social and cultural analyses of the meaning and significance of opioids in American society, and therefore I will not undertake such analysis.

But given the centrality of opioids in the PPSG approach, as well as the undeniable fact that opioids remain an important intervention in treating pain, this book would be incomplete if it did not at least briefly address some of the issues swirling around the use and abuse of opioid analgesics. Consistent with the ethos of this book, my chief interest is in the ways that the meaning of opioids in American society is reflected in opioid policy.

OPIOIDS AND THE MEANING OF
ADDICTION IN AMERICAN SOCIETY

Pain scholars frequently argue that the undertreatment of pain is inextricably intertwined with the undermedication of pain.[21] Morris focuses on acute pain resultant to terminal illness perhaps in part because of the "bitter irony that in almost all cases effective medications are available but not used."[22] He acknowledges that physician fears regarding possible addiction to opiates drive undermedication, but is also aware that fears about opioids permeate society in general, and are shared by the pain sufferers themselves, who are often "no less wary of opiates and opioids than are many doctors."[23] Nessa Coyle's 2004 study of terminally ill cancer patients revealed that virtually all of them expressed great concern over opioid therapy, voicing anxiety that the side effects of opioids would "make them sleepy or dull their minds."[24] One patient could not "countenance" the possibility that both his increasing pain and his increasing sensation of being "zonked out" "were associated with progressive disease *as well as* opioid side effects. . . ."[25]

Although many pain scholars had for decades argued that the risks of addiction are extremely small,[26] given the striking increase in fatalities connected to prescription drug use, such conclusions are subject to increasing skepticism. However, while concerns of addiction and prescription drug misuse may be warranted, two other common fears that attend the use of opioids may be less justified: respiratory depression and tolerance. The best evidence suggests that the probability of these effects occurring as a result of the use of opioids is much lower than had been surmised, to the point that withholding otherwise indicated opioids for these reasons is generally suboptimal if not substandard care.[27]

Even assuming that the fears of addiction, respiratory depression, and tolerance are entirely unjustified, there is reason to suspect that explaining as such to prescribers and patients may do little to dislodge those who hold these views. This is all the more true with a highly publicized fear attending opioid prescription, that of criminal prosecution.

CRIMINAL PROSECUTION FOR OPIOIDS

There is vigorous debate over the extent of the risk of criminal prosecution for opioids. For at least two decades, numerous books and articles on the subject have been produced, and the contest shows no signs of diminishing. In 2008, an article appeared in the prominent journal *Pain Medicine* analyzing the "big picture" regarding the nature and characteristics of both criminal prosecution and administrative enforcement (generally actions taken by state medical boards against prescribers).[28] The authors found that only 0.1 percent of prescribers between 1998 and 2006 experienced either criminal prosecution or administrative action, and concluded that both criminal and administrative enforcement activity was rare.[29] The authors also noted that their data did not suggest that pain specialists faced any increased risk of enforcement activity.[30] The article ignited a storm of controversy. Among those involved in the fray was political scientist Ronald T. Libby, the author of a book entitled *The Criminalization of Medicine: America's War on Doctors*.[31] Libby maintains that the risks of enforcement activity are quite real, so much so that they amount to a virtual "war" on opioid prescribers, and he referred to several "serious and obvious flaws in the research" covered in the Goldenbaum et al. study.[32]

Of course, it is unlikely that an academic article could merit such media attention without several high-profile criminal prosecutions of pain physicians during the last few years. Arguably, the most visible of these cases are the trials of William Hurwitz, a pain physician prosecuted by the federal government for narcotics trafficking. Hurwitz was originally convicted in 2004 and was sentenced to 28 years in prison, but prevailed on appeal.[33] The government won again on retrial, and in 2007, Hurwitz was sentenced to serve 57 months in prison. The Hurwitz case evoked extensive coverage from all manner of stakeholders interested in the treatment of pain. Numerous pain advocacy organizations, professional societies, and editors of relevant journals followed the case closely, many of whom expressed heated reactions to Hurwitz's second conviction and incarceration.

There are two overarching points I want to make regarding criminal prosecution for opioids. First, in a very real sense it makes little difference whether those who claim that the risks of enforcement activity for opioid prescribing are small or their adversaries are correct. This is because the fears of enforcement are quite real. Regardless of the absolute risks, the fact remains that prescribers of opioid analgesics maintain such fears. As such, telling those prescribers that their fears are unwarranted may do little to dispel them. In an editorial accompanying the Goldenbaum et al. study, pain scholar Sandra Johnson noted that the "consistent evidence-based message" that the risks of enforcement are small "cannot compete with the grapevine and news headlines of the horror story."[34]

Moreover, Judge Learned Hand's seminal formula for assessing negligence notes that what matters in thinking about what the reasonably prudent person would do is not simply the probability of the harm occurring, but that probability multiplied by the magnitude of the harm that could occur.[35] Johnson observes that prescribers' fears may track Hand's insight, because while the "incidence may be rare," the injury, if it were to occur, would be "great" indeed.[36] Finally, Johnson notes the abundant social science research demonstrating that

> debunking false information actually contributes to its persistence. People who hear information they believe is true—for example, that prescribing controlled substances for pain is risky—and then hear multiple times that the information is actually false are more likely to remember the false information as true than are those individuals who do not hear the multiple refutations.[37]

The point is that, while not quite irrelevant, precisely calibrating the risks opioid prescribers face of enforcement activity is of secondary importance where prescribers do in fact fear such enforcement activity. Informing prescribers that their fears are out of proportion to the risks may do little to dispel such fears. If Johnson is correct, a constant flow of information suggesting the disproportion of the fears may actually *intensify* them.[38] A preferable means of proceeding, then, is to focus less on specifying the nature of the risk prescribers face, and instead to attempt an understanding of the meaning of the fears. Why do prescribers fear prosecution or administrative action for prescribing opioids? Note that this question is a corollary of the question that the PPSG's focus on balance in opioid policy implies but does not answer: why is it that opioid policy in the U.S. has historically been imbalanced?

One other example will hopefully suffice to demonstrate the importance of unpacking the meaning of opioids and addiction in American society in producing ethical opioid policies that address the root causes of such imbalance. In the retrial of William Hurwitz, the government introduced as one of its expert witnesses Robin Hamill-Ruth, a pain medicine physician and the Director of the Pain Management Center at University of Virginia Health Systems.[39] Upon cross-examination, defense counsel questioned Hamill-Ruth regarding the care of a chronic pain patient named Kathleen Lohrey.[40] Lohrey suffered from severe, debilitating migraines, and sought relief at the Pain Management Center Hamill-Ruth directed, but, according to the *New York Times,* found to her dismay that the "clinic's philosophy 'includes avoidance of all opioids in chronic headache management.'" Given the evidence suggesting that opioids may be an effective treatment for at least some persons who suffer from chronic head pain,[42] the question is what would prompt a center devoted to treating pain to disavow the use of an evidence-based intervention? The phenomenology of pain is crucial here; Kathleen Lohrey abandoned Hamill-Ruth's pain clinic in despair and frustration after she was prescribed buspirone, an anti-anxiolytic drug whose known side effects include headaches.[43] After receiving opioid prescriptions from Hurwitz, she testified as a witness in his defense.

In any case, the question remains: why did the pain clinic expressly state as its philosophy that it would generally avoid treating headaches with opioid analgesics? Any answer to this question that does not include an analysis of the meaning of opioids in American culture is hopelessly flawed.

THE MEANING OF OPIOIDS

Fears of addiction attending the use of opioids are not novel. The renowned medieval physician Guy de Chauliac warned as such during the fourteenth century, and the risks of addiction were well understood in the early modern era as well.[44] Nevertheless, there is no question that the issue took on particular importance in the nineteenth century, with the advent of anesthesia and the Victorian focus on the general relief of suffering and pain.

Perhaps the most intriguing aspect of this period is the fact that fear of pharmaceutical analgesics was readily apparent virtually from the inception of modern anesthesia itself. Pernick notes that "in mid-nineteenth-century America, humane, conscientious, highly reputable practitioners and ordinary lay people held many misgivings about the new discovery."[45] This comment underscores another reason for preferring an approach to pain that goes beyond opioid policy: a focus only on the gatekeepers for opioid dispensation risks casting the prescribers into a hero/villain dichotomy. It is reasonable to presume that the majority of prescribers do not wish ill upon their patients, and that the reasons why pain is undertreated are only poorly correlated, if at all, with the existence of vicious prescribers. Morris concurs, noting that "[b]laming doctors as inhumane just won't work."[46]

There were very real drawbacks to the use of anesthesia in mid-nineteenth-century America. On the technical level, very little was known about anesthesia, so it was difficult if not impossible to determine safe dosage levels.[47] Chloroform, for example, has proven to have a panoply of dangerous side effects. Anesthesia itself is inherently dangerous, as "[t]he administration of anesthesia necessarily involves some practices and procedures that might be viewed as 'resuscitation' in other settings."[48] As such, anesthesiologists have generally voiced concern over do-not-resuscitate orders, fearing legitimately that without careful wording, such orders could be construed to prohibit the typical resuscitative measures that attend the use of general anesthesia.[49]

To handle these issues, nineteenth-century healers typically undertook what Pernick terms a "calculus of professionalism" in which the healer queried which was the " 'lesser evil'—the harm likely to be caused by the pain or the harm that might be caused by the painkiller?"[50] Yet Pernick cautions that "the strength and longevity of nineteenth-century fears about the safety of anesthesia cannot be explained simply by the fact that modern medicine shares some of these concerns."[51] Indeed, the calculus at issue was both moral and clinical; the question of which "evil" was morally worse deeply influenced healing practices of the time.

The point is that the fear that the cure for pain is worse than the 'disease' is hardly a novel phenomenon. It has its roots in the earliest attitudes to modern anesthesia. Hill suggests that such attitudes are "systematically transferred from one generation of physicians to another,"[52] which reflects an appropriately dialectic model of history. In such a model, prior events, ideas, and conditions shape current attitudes and beliefs. Understanding current fears about opioids and addiction therefore benefits from a culturally and historically informed understanding of traditional fears about medical interventions used to ameliorate pain.

Central to Pernick's analysis is the notion that the treatment of pain needed and dispensed through opioids varied depending on the demographic and social characteristics of the person in pain. It was widely believed that African-Americans had much higher pain thresholds than white persons.[53] Indeed, this belief was the primary justification J. Marion Sims offered for conducting his vesicovaginal fistula experiments on black slaves as opposed to some of his more well-heeled (white) patients.[54] The current evidence regarding the scope of inequities in assessing and treating pain suggests there are some important links between the history of opioids in the nineteenth century and current attitudes, practices, and beliefs related to the use of opioids.[55]

Furthermore, the concept of addiction must itself be historicized. Joseph Gabriel has documented how the concept of addiction itself is a peculiarly twentieth-century phenomenon.[56] Challenging the notion that drugs themselves are purely biological entities, Gabriel argues that

> [t]he fact that the physical drug that is put in the body is itself constituted through the processes of agriculture, pharmaceutical research, and manufacturing—which are themselves constituted through various hybrid forces that partake of both the material and cultural aspects of the world—means that drug chemistry is no more outside of human culture than any other aspect of the drug experience.[57]

He continues by arguing that while addiction "obviously did not exist before people started consuming certain types of commodities . . . it also did not exist before people started understanding themselves in terms of the binary between autonomy and self-discipline on the one hand and a lack of self-control and bondage on the other."[58] While opium, hashish, ether, morphine, and cocaine were "used therapeutically before becoming sites of social panic . . . by the end of the nineteenth century . . . the consumption of these substances outside of direct medical supervision had become an area of profound concern for doctors and pharmacists."[59] Similarly, historian of addiction Caroline Acker notes that the idea of the 'American junkie' is a twentieth-century construction.[60]

The notion that addiction itself has a history, and would have been poorly understood, if at all, even by habitual 'users' of opioids and other 'dangerous' drugs in the nineteenth century is crucial in making sense of contemporary fears of addiction. Properly historicizing addiction does not require denying the reality of addiction or suggesting that fears of opioid addiction are irrational. Rather, a responsible historical approach locates such fears in context, and suggests some of the deeply entrenched social and cultural reasons why so many prescribers and pain sufferers alike fear the power and the apparent danger of opioids.

Notwithstanding the importance of this meaning to understanding the historical imbalance in opioid policy and some of the fears providers, pain sufferers, and caregivers share with respect to opioids, the meaning of opioids and addiction is not coextensive with the meaning of pain. Moreover, undue focus on the meaning of opioids and addiction seems to suggest a policy focus on opioid regulation, which is a direction I do not endorse for the reasons detailed in this chapter.

The following chapter is devoted to detailing and justifying the policy directions I do endorse as to pain. I demonstrate how these policy recommendations incorporate the social and cultural evidence I have adduced, as well as the ethical imperative to center the pain sufferer, and justify a hope that, if implemented, improvement in the culture of pain is possible.

NOTES

1. The literature on this topic is immense. For a helpful introduction, see the NIH Roadmap for Translational Research, last accessed Jan. 8, 2009, from http://nihroadmap.nih.gov/.
2. See The Institute of Medicine, *The Future of the Public's Health in the 21st Century* (Washington, DC: National Academies Press, 2002).
3. Gilson, Joranson, Ryan, Maurer, Moen, and Kline, *Achieving Balance in Federal and State Pain Policy*, § V.
4. Ibid.
5. Goldberg, "The Sole Indexicality of Pain."
6. Acker, *Creating the American Junkie;* and Acker, "From All Purposes Anodyne to Marker of Deviance."
7. Stratton Hill, Jr., personal communication to author, 2009.
8. Richard DeGrandpre, *The Cult of Pharmacology: How America Became the World's most Troubled Drug Culture* (Durham, NC: Duke University Press, 2006)

9. In addition, there has been extensive concern over the connections between the PPSG and associated pain advocacy groups such as the American Pain Foundation ("APF") and the pharmaceutical industry. The ties between the groups prompted Senator Charles Grassley (R—Iowa) to initiate an investigation into the relationships and flows of funding. Inasmuch as the efforts of the PPSG and the APF helped facilitate the general liberalization of opioid utilization in the U.S., said efforts obviously align with the interests of pharmaceutical drug manufacturers that produce opioid analgesics. In May 2012, the American Pain Foundation officially dissolved. See Charles Ornstein and Tracy Weber, "American Pain Foundation Shuts Down as Senators Launch Investigation of Prescription Narcotics," accessed February 26, 2013, from http://www.propublica.org/article/senate-panel-investigates-drug-company-ties-to-pain-groups. Analysis of these conflicts-of-interest is reserved for future work.

10. Amol Deshpande, Andrea D. Furlan, Angela Mailis-Gagnon, Steven Atlas, and Denis Turk, "Opioids for Chronic Low Back Pain," *Cochrane Database of Systematic Reviews* 3, Art. No.: CD004959 (July 2007), doi:10.1002/14651858.CD004959.pub3, accessed June 1, 2009, from http://dx.doi.org/10.1002/14651858.CD004959.pub3 (citation omitted).

11. Jane C Ballantyne, "Medical Use of Opioids: What Drives the Debate? A Brief Commentary," *European Journal of Pain Supplements* 2, no. 1 (October 2008): 67–8.

12. Deshpande, Furlan, Mailis-Gagnon, Atlas, and Turk, "Opioids for Chronic Low Back Pain," 13.

13. Meredith Noble, Stephen J. Tregear, Jonathan R. Treadwell, and Karen Schoelles, "Long-Term Opioid Therapy for Chronic Noncancer Pain: A Systematic Review and Meta-Analysis of Efficacy and Safety," *Journal of Pain and Symptom Management* 35, no. 2 (February 2008): 222. A more recent systematic review produced by many of the same authors noted exactly the same conclusion, that only "weak evidence suggests that patients who are able to continue opioids long-term experience clinically significant pain relief." Meredith Noble, Jonathan R. Treadwell, Stephen J. Tregear, Vivian H. Coates, Phillip J. Wiffen, Clarisse Akafomo, and Karen M. Scholles, "Long-Term Opioid Management for Chronic Noncancer Pain," *Cochrane Database of Systematic Reviews* 11, Art. No.: CD006605 (2010), doi:10.1002/14651858.CD006605.pub2, from http://dx.doi.org/10.1002/14651858.CD006605.pub2.

14. Deshpande, Furlan, Mailis-Gagnon, Atlas, and Turk, "Opioids for Chronic Low-Back Pain," 13.

15. For more on the idea that there exist multiple phenomenologies of pain, see the Preface and Chapter 2 (this volume).

16. E.g., Carol A. Warfield and Zahid H. Bajwa, *Principles and Practice of Pain Medicine*, 2nd ed. (New York, NY: McGraw Hill Companies, 2004).

17. Chapter 7 (this volume) discusses the role of touch, including massage, as therapy for pain.

18. E.g., Denise O'Connor, Shawn C. Marshall, and Nicola Massy-Westropp, "Non-Surgical Treatment (Other Than Steroid Injection) for Carpal Tunnel Syndrome," *Cochrane Database of Systematic Reviews* 1, Art. No.: CD003219 (January 2003), doi:10.1002/14651858.CD003219, accessed June 12, 2009, from http://dx.doi.org/10.1002/14651858.CD003219.

19. Christopher Eccleston, Amanda C de C Williams, and Stephen Morley, "Psychological Therapies for the Management of Chronic Pain (Excluding Headache) in Adults," *Cochrane Database of Systematic Reviews,* 2, Art. No.: CD007407 (April 2009), doi:10.1002/14651858.CD007407.pub2, accessed June 13, 2009, from http://dx.doi.org/10.1002/14651858.CD007407.pub2.

20. Won, Lapane, Vallow, Schein, Morris, and Lipsitz, "Persistent Nonmalignant Pain and Analgesic Prescribing Patterns in Elderly Nursing Home Residents"; Teno, Weitzen, Wetle, and Mor, "Persistent Pain in Nursing Home Residents"; and Ferrell, Ferrell, and Rivera, "Pain in Cognitively Impaired Nursing Home Patients."

21. E.g., Morris, "An Invisible History of Pain"; Ben A. Rich, "An Ethical Analysis of the Barriers to Effective Pain Management," *Cambridge Quarterly of Health Care Ethics* 9, no. 1 (January 2000): 54–70; Ben A. Rich, "A Legacy of Silence: Bioethics and the Culture of Pain," *Journal of Medical Humanities* 18, no. 4 (December 1997): 233–59.

22. Morris, *Illness and Culture in the Postmodern Age*, 113.

23. Ibid.

24. Nessa Coyle, "In Their Own Words: Seven Advanced Cancer Patients Describe Their Experience with Pain and the Use of Opioid Drugs," *Journal of Pain and Symptom Management* 27, no. 4 (April 2004): 304–5.

25. Ibid.

26. Morris, *Illness and Culture in the Postmodern Age*, 107–34.

27. Consensus Statement of the American Academy of Pain Medicine and the American Pain Society, accessed June16, 2009, from http://www.ampainsoc. org/advocacy/opioids.htm.

28. Donald M. Goldenbaum, Myra Christopher, Rollin M. Gallagher, Scott Fishman, Richard Payne, David Joranson, Drew Edmondson, Judith McKee, and Arthur Thexton, "Physicians Charged with Opioid Analgesic-Prescribing Offenses," *Pain Medicine* 9, no. 6 (September 2008): 737–47.

29. Ibid.

30. Ibid.

31. Ronald T. Libby, *The Criminalization of Medicine: America's War on Doctors* (Westport, CT: Greenwood Publishing Group, 2007).

32. Ronald T. Libby, e-mail message to author, September 27, 2008.

33. *United States v. Hurwitz*, 459 F.3d 363 (4th Cir. 2006).

34. Sandra H. Johnson, "Editorial," *Pain Medicine* 9, no. 6 (September 2008): 748–9.

35. Learned Hand is one of the most famous judges in American history. He authored his formula for negligence in the case of *United States v. Carroll Towing Co.*, 159 F.2d 169 (2d Cir. 1947). The formula is written as B <pL, where B is the burden of the act needed to prevent the harm, p is the probability of the harm occurring, and L is the magnitude of the harm were it to occur. Where the burden of acting is lower than the probability of the harm multiplied by its magnitude, the actor's failure to act accordingly constitutes negligence. The reasonable doubts as to whether the concept of negligence can be formalized in this way should not prevent the reader from grasping the utility of Hand's frame in thinking through some of the moral and legal implications of risk.

36. Sandra H. Johnson, "Editorial," *Pain Medicine* 9, no. 6 (2008): 748.

37. Ibid., 749.

38. Norbert Schwarz, Lawrence J. Sanna, Ian Skurnik, and Carolyn Yoon, "Metacognitive Experiences and the Intricacies of Setting People Straight: Implications for Debiasing and Public Information Campaigns," *Advances in Experimental Social Psychology* 39, ed. Mark Zanna (New York, NY: Academic Press, 2007), 127–61; Kimberlee Weaver, Stephen M. Garcia, Norbert Schwarz, and Dale T. Miller, "Inferring the Popularity of an Opinion From Its Familiarity: A Repetitive Voice Can Sound Like a Chorus," *Journal of Personality and Social Psychology* 92, no. 5 (May 2007): 821–33.

39. John Tierney, "At Trial, Pain has a Witness," *New York Times*, April 24, 2007.

40. Ibid.

41. Ibid.

42. Dewey K. Ziegler, "Opioids In Headache Treatment: Is There a Role?" *Neurologic Clinics* 15, no. 1 (February 1997): 199–207. In a longitudinal study of clinical efficacy of daily scheduled opioids for intractable head pain, Joel R. Saper et al. noted that while a select group of the subjects (26 percent, n = 41) benefited considerably from the regimen, the remaining 74 percent (n = 119) either failed to show improvement or were discontinued from the program for clinical reasons. Therefore, again it is important in discussing the use of opioids for treating pain to understand that the effectiveness of such treatments for any particular type of pain remains unsettled. Joel R. Saper, Alvin E. Lake III, Robert L. Hamel, Thomas E. Lutz, Barbaranne Branca, Dorothy B. Sims, and Mary M. Kroll, "Daily Scheduled Opioids for Intractable Head Pain: Long Term Observations of a Treatment Program," *Neurology* 62, no. 10 (May 25, 2004): 1687–94.

43. For an excellent introduction into some of the historical issues surrounding the treatment of headaches in the U.S., see Jan R. McTavish, *Pain & Profits: The History of the Headache and Its Remedies in America* (New Brunswick, NJ: Rutgers University Press, 2004).

44. See Silverman, *Tortured Subjects*.

45. Pernick, *A Calculus of Suffering*, 35.

46. Morris, *Illness and Culture in the Postmodern Age*, 195–6.

47. Pernick, *A Calculus of Suffering*.

48. American Society of Anesthesiologists, "Ethical Guidelines for the Anesthesia Care of Patients with Do-Not-Resuscitate Orders," accessed June 16, 2009, from http://www.asahq.org/publicationsAndServices/standards/09.html.

49. Ibid.

50. Pernick, *A Calculus of Suffering*, 95.

51. Ibid., 39.

52. Hill, "When Will Adequate Pain Management be the Norm," 1881.

53. Pernick, *A Calculus of Suffering*.

54. Ibid; Caroline M. De Costa, "James Marion Sims: Some Speculations and a New Position," *The Medical Journal of Australia* 178, no. 12 (June 16, 2003): 660–3.

55. For a brief analysis of this connection as to elderly patients, see Goldberg, "The Sole Indexicality of Pain."

56. Gabriel, "Gods and Monsters.

57. Ibid., 9.

58. Ibid., 10.

59. Ibid., 14.

60. Acker, *Creating the American Junkie*.

8 Evidence-Based Pain Policy Recommendations

INTRODUCTION

Crafting public health policy is difficult. One reason for its difficulty is Deborah Stone's admonition that policy is inevitably contested space.[1] Even seemingly innocuous policies require a trade-off of time and resources invested in their production, pursuit, and implementation. This means that the justification for any proposed policy must be robust, and the rhetoric employed in the justification is crucial.[2] This notion of rhetoric suggests the second important lesson: because policy and politics are inextricably linked, and because the political process involves myriad stakeholders with myriad interests and concerns, building the relationships needed to produce, pursue, and implement desired policy requires the utilization of rhetoric and arguments that are responsive to the interests of the particular audience(s).[3]

Between 2007 and 2010, I served as Chief Policy Advisor on a grant-funded health inequalities research project that brought together over 300 collaborators drawn from public, private, and nonprofit community-based sectors. To guide this diverse network, the project leaders and I, with the assistance of several process consultants, produced a list of "Policy Process Questions."[4] The work required to answer these questions essentially provided both the rationale and the general form of the policy recommendations themselves, which were then revised and edited numerous times before being released. The two lessons mentioned above—the notion of policy as a contest and the importance of tailoring rhetoric to suit the interests of the audience—were instrumental in shaping these Policy Process Questions:

1. What is the problem? How does it manifest itself?
2. What would success look like? (Goal)
3. Whose behavior needs to change in order to achieve the goal? (Target Audience)
4. Who has the ability to change the behavior of the target audience? (Political Actor)

   5. What policy is recommended to achieve the behavior change in the target audience? (Ignore perceived limitations)
   6. What is the feasibility of this policy?
   7. What are potential unintended consequences of this policy?
   8. What are some primary social, political, ethical, financial obstacles to implementing this policy?
   9. What is the underlying thinking on why this policy will be effective?

The questions that seemed to prompt the most confusion were numbers 3 and 4. These questions are also the most significant steps, because they required the participants to apprehend the crucial difference between those actors whose behavior the policies are intended to change and those actors and entities who enjoy the power needed to actually implement the recommended policies. If, for example, it is physicians whose behavior a given health policy is intended to change, targeting the language of the policy only to individual physicians guarantees that it will accomplish little, because individual physicians generally do not find themselves in a position to implement broad-based health policy.

This is not to imply there is no value in a recommendation geared to individual physicians, but rather that such a recommendation more closely resembles a position statement than a broad-based health policy. Asserting that individual physicians ought to do X may be a perfectly plausible position to adopt, but there is a very great difference between adopting a position and producing a policy with the hope that it could be implemented. If in fact the proposed policy is intended to change practices of individual physicians, the actors or entities that maintain the capacity to do so are, from a policy perspective, the prime audience. Depending on the specific policy in question, examples of such actors include professional societies such as the American Medical Association or the American College of Surgeons, the American Association of Medical Colleges (which exerts a strong influence on medical education), or the Centers for Medicare & Medicaid Services (CMS), the federal agency that determines Medicare and (the federal component of) Medicaid reimbursement policy.

Thus, an optimal health policy is neither too general nor too specific. If the proposed policy is too general, it runs the risk of appearing to be a position statement that is not closely tied to the audience possessing the capacity to effect change. If the proposed policy is too specific, it runs the risk of having only a narrow impact, limiting the potential reach and signaling effect of the policy even before it is implemented.

The Policy Process Questions are neither formula nor algorithm. Rather, they are simply a guide, a rough heuristic incorporating some of these key policy points. The bulk of this chapter is devoted to determining whether they will be of any use as applied to the undertreatment of pain.

PAIN AND THE POLICY PROCESS

Question #1: What Is the Problem? How Does It Manifest?

The problem is the undertreatment of pain. It manifests in myriad health care encounters in which a person seeks treatment of their pain, or presents with health problems that include pain. Such encounters are not limited to visits to a doctor's office, but include a number of different situations in which illness is assessed and treated and care provided (for example, long-term care facilities, ambulatory clinics, emergency rooms, etc.).

In the vast majority of these encounters, health care providers and entities possess the technical capacity to treat the pain effectively. Chapter 1 (this volume) shows that in far too many of these encounters, pain is either not treated at all or is not treated effectively. In addition, the treatment that is provided is dispensed along various social fault lines such as race, class, gender, and age, and inequities in pain are a significant and growing problem.

Question #2: What Would Success Look Like? (Goal)

Success in the undertreatment of pain most obviously and most directly looks like an American society in which pain is treated commensurate with the technical proficiency available. In this hypothetical society, inequities in the assessment and treatment of pain are decreasing, and vulnerable and marginalized populations are the recipients of increased focus and resources as to the assessment and treatment of pain.

However, such objectives are not the only markers of success. Better and more equitable treatment of pain may be the ultimate goals, but are only tenable if facilitated by a different, more virtuous "culture of pain" in American society. The idea of a "culture of pain" received its most extensive treatment in David Morris's 1991 book, but recognition of its significance is growing. The IOM's 2011 report calls for a "cultural transformation" as to the treatment of pain, but does little to specify what such a transformation would look like. I believe that the most important criterion of an improved culture of pain is whether the pain sufferer's lived, subjective experiences are centered by providers, caregivers, and sufferers alike. A society in which the pain sufferer's experiences were the primary focus in any pain encounter would reflect a culture of pain in which its effective treatment is more likely and more equitable. I will say more about the culture of pain below.

Question #3: Whose Behavior Needs to Change in Order to Achieve the Goal? (Target Audience)

One of my central claims has been that the meaning of pain is a dynamic, ever-changing product of the interactions of a number of different stakeholders.

I have expressly criticized approaches to the problem of undertreated pain that focus on only one of these key agents, typically the provider, and even more typically, the physician. As important as the provider and the physician are to improving the culture of pain, it is not only providers whose practices need to change to improve the undertreatment of pain. I have noted multiple times that elderly populations in the U.S. tend to underreport their pain, at times substantially so. This tendency is a barrier to the effective treatment of members of this population. It is uncomfortable on a variety of levels to suggest that changing some aspects of pain sufferers' behavior could produce a more virtuous culture of pain, at least in part because it seems to imply a blame-the-victim mentality, that pain sufferers bear responsibility for their pain.[5] Given the intense stigma that pain sufferers face in the U.S., it would be a grievous sin indeed to imply that such alienation is self-inflicted.

Let me be as clear as possible: pain sufferers are neither culpable for their pain nor do they deserve to suffer it while safe and effective remedies exist. This conclusion simply does not follow from the premise that pain sufferers themselves are active participants in a discourse that tends to deemphasize and delegitimize the lived experiences of pain. What does follow is that socialization is inordinately powerful. The social and cultural narratives and conceptualizations of objectivity, the power of the visible, and the relationship between the mind and the body that shape American attitudes, practices, and beliefs towards the meaning of pain are deeply rooted. As such, it should not be surprising that these deep-seeded conceptualizations frame the understandings of pain sufferers themselves.

Centering the pain sufferer does not imply that the role of the pain sufferer is simply to teach the other participants in the culture of pain. Quite the contrary, teaching and learning are connected. There is no reason that pain sufferers cannot both teach others about their lived experiences of pain and learn about the ways, subtle and otherwise, in which American society tends to decenter such experiences. Such learning can and should include information related to the ways in which even pain sufferers' behaviors can contribute to such decentering.

So, whose behavior needs to change? Principally providers, caregivers, and pain sufferers, and likely in that order of importance.

Question #4a: Who Has the Ability to Change the Behavior of the Target Audience? (Political Actor)

Recall again the difference between questions #3 and #4. The actors whose behavior needs to change are frequently not identical to the actors and entities that have the ability to change the relevant behaviors. Thus, if it is principally the behavior and ways of understanding pain among providers, caregivers, and pain sufferers that should change, who or what enjoys the capacity to influence each of these actors' practices and conceptions as to pain?

As to health care providers, the answer depends, of course, on which providers we identify as relevant. Physicians, to be sure, but not simply physicians: among others, nurses, physician assistants, psychologists, social workers, and allied health professionals are also involved in treating persons in pain. What stakeholders maintain the capacity to change behavior of all of these different professionals? Answers to question #4 often converge on the merits of working both from the top-down and from the bottom-up. This resolution reflects the idea that while large and powerful actors often exert a significant effect on practices, at the same time, our social worlds are inevitably local, and thus a great deal of what shapes and informs habits and practices are correspondingly local.

While there are several suitable actors that are well-positioned to exert a top-down influence on the practices and conceptions of providers, the most appropriate in the U.S. is CMS. This is primarily because CMS sets federal reimbursement policy for Medicare and Medicaid. Given that in 2010 Medicare funds alone represented approximately 3.6 percent of U.S. GDP (roughly $440 billion),[6] a proportion that is unlikely to decrease with the implementation of the Affordable Care Act ("ACA"),[7] reimbursement policy is a powerful tool indeed in regulating behaviors of those actors who rely on federal reimbursement.

Many different kinds of health care providers, of course, are so reliant, but so too are the vast majority of hospitals, whether for-profit or non-profit, and health care entities as defined under applicable federal and state laws. Though a growing number of providers and entities are refusing to provide care to any person covered by a third-party payer, it nevertheless remains true that Medicare reimbursement remains a crucial axis through which health care is delivered and financed in the U.S. The undeniable fact that Medicare is a linchpin throughout the currently fragmented, discombobulated structure of health care in the U.S. is not lost on the federal government, which wields the power to limit or bar entities from participating in the Medicare program as a sword to regulate all manner of conduct.[8] So too do private actors like the Joint Commission rely on this sword; hospitals and health care entities that satisfy the Joint Commission accreditation standards are deemed to qualify for participation in the Medicare program,[9] which is as powerful a financial incentive as exists to ensure compliance.

However, the impact of CMS policy is not limited solely to those whose livelihood depends on federal reimbursement. Private third-party payers such as managed care organizations typically incorporate significant portions of CMS reimbursement policy into their own coverage determinations,[10] which means that CMS policy exerts a significant impact even on providers who do not rely on federal reimbursement.

Ultimately, there is good justification for thinking that CMS is a prime actor capable of utilizing its reimbursement power to regulate behavior that operates at a level substantially downstream from CMS itself. With a suitable actor identified, the analysis can move on to policy process question #5:

Question #5a: What Policy Is Recommended to Achieve the Behavior Change in the Target Audience? (Ignore Perceived Limitations)

I designate this question #5a because different policies will obviously be needed to accompany the different actors that possess the capacity to change the behavior (question #4) of the different target audiences (question #3). So, as to CMS, what policy is recommended to achieve the behavior change? The answer to this question constitutes Pain Policy Recommendation #1:

PAIN POLICY RECOMMENDATION #1

Because centering the pain sufferer is crucial to improving the undertreatment of pain, CMS should amend its reimbursement structure so as to provide maximum coverage for time spent listening to the patient.

At some level, this recommendation seems absurdly simple, even naïve. With all of the urgent problems plaguing the delivery and financing of health care in the U.S., the first policy recommendation as to improving the treatment of pain is simply to encourage *listening* to the patient? The answer to this question is an emphatic "yes."

First, there is excellent evidence that listening to illness sufferers is a skill in short supply in American health care.[11] There are many reasons for this, though one of the most significant is the focus I have identified on the objects that cause disease in place of attention to the illness sufferer him or herself. As explained in detail in chapters 2–4 (this volume), the imperative to engage the illness sufferer's lifeworld and listen to his/her stories and experiences lessens as the clinical gaze rises in importance to medicine and healing during the nineteenth century. Where the primary (exciting) cause of the illness sufferer's diptheria is identified as a cornyebacterium, and where a specific antitoxin is available, the importance of engaging the sufferer's subjective life to determine which permutation of conditions, events, and habits converge to produce illness recedes.

The theme of this book is that the pain sufferer's subjective, lived experiences must be centered. This, of course, is intended as a counter to the objectifying tendencies of Western (American) culture in general and of the American culture of biomedicine in particular. The particular, local lifeworld of the pain sufferer must occupy pride of place in clinical pain encounters if any improvement in the treatment of pain and the culture of pain in which treatment practices are situated is to be expected. Moreover, listening to the illness sufferer is obviously at the core of cognitive behavioral therapy (though such therapy just as obviously involves a great deal more than listening), an intervention that is safe and effective in treating some kinds of chronic pain.

Finally, I have noted the evidence suggesting that communication between pain sufferers and providers is poor. Jackson believes that relationships between chronic pain sufferers and physicians are the worst in American health care, with high levels of mutual mistrust and frequent and inequitable stigma directed at chronic pain sufferers.[12] It is therefore not difficult to understand why improving the capacity of providers to listen to and engage the lifeworld of their patients, to hear the sufferers' lived experiences of pain, would almost certainly improve the culture of pain, and thereby facilitate improved treatment of pain.[13]

The reason this imperative is served by the recommendation regarding CMS is the fact that the problems in listening are exacerbated by Medicare reimbursement policy.[14] Medicare, like the vast majority of health care institutions in the U.S., reflects the acute care paradigm on which it was modeled.[15] Medicare is essentially a fee-for-service program, which suggests that it tends to reimburse discrete, identifiable tasks associated with acute care episodes relatively well.[16] Despite the fact that Medicare, because of its roots in traditional fee-for-service indemnity, is ill-suited to caring for chronic illness sufferers, "the Medicare program is in reality a program serving people with chronic conditions—typically, multiple chronic conditions—for whom traditional indemnity insurance principles and coverage are not appropriate and whose health status presents a challenge for both cost and quality of care."[17] Wagner et al. documented in 2001 "growing discrepancies between current reimbursement policies of the Centers for Medicare and Medicaid Services . . . and private insurers and interventions shown to improve chronic disease care."[18]

The procedure-based system of reimbursement Medicare produces all sorts of deleterious effects, most of which have been documented by a group at Dartmouth Medical School, who have for the last several decades documented how a staggering percentage of Medicare funds have been expended on interventions that are not evidence-based and that have had no discernible impact on either morbidity or mortality.[19]

As to pain, an additional side effect of Medicare's fee-for-service nature is that time spent communicating with and listening to the illness sufferer generally does not qualify as a discrete "service" under applicable federal guidelines. This means that time and resources expended on simply speaking with and listening to the illness sufferer are either not reimbursed at all, or are reimbursed at lower levels and with greater uncertainty of expected reimbursement.[20] Thus, the general social and cultural narratives in American culture and in the culture of American biomedicine that tend to discourage listening to and engaging the lifeworld of the pain sufferer are exacerbated by a Medicare reimbursement structure that provides financial disincentives for doing so (because time spent listening to a patient is time not spent on optimally reimbursable services). Discrete clinical services used in treating (acute) visible, material pathologies tend to be maximally reimbursable under Medicare; listening to the pain sufferer tends to receive much lower levels of reimbursement.

Of course, the fact that Medicare reimbursement policy discourages listening to the patient is unsurprising given the power and impact of the American emphasis on greater abstraction, greater objectification, and greater quantification in medicine and science.[21] This too underscores the idea that a given legal and regulatory regime is itself a product of culture.

Nevertheless, the fact that such a reimbursement scheme should not be unexpected given the role objectification plays in American culture does not imply that it is ethically acceptable. Given the scope and impact of CMS policy on providers and entities across and within American health care, there is reason to suspect that a superior reimbursement structure, one that encouraged rather than impeded the process of listening to the pain sufferer, could have a salutary effect on the culture of pain and could thereby facilitate better treatment of pain.

Admittedly, I am not the first to issue such a recommendation. In urging a turn to what he terms "narrative bioethics," David Morris argues that a concept of clinically effective listening has significant ethical important for actual practice.[22] This follows insofar as refusing to listen to what others say is an expression of utmost disrespect.[23] Morris concludes with what for him is a remarkably stark judgment: "Doctors who neglect to gain the skills and knowledge required for clinically effective listening—although this idea is absolutely foreign to Western medicine—are engaged in unethical medical practice."[24] Similarly, in a 2005 essay, Rita Charon, one of the leading practitioners, scholars, and educators of what she originally termed "narrative medicine," specifically addressed the capacity of the kind of close listening that attention to texts and narratives can encourage in context of pain. Charon argues that narrative is particularly required by patients with chronic pain because "[w]ords are often all the patient has."[25] Conversely, health care providers that treat people in pain need narrative competence because treating complex pain conditions requires partnership and an authenticity of self that facility with pain sufferers' stories can help build.[26] But although the call has been issued, there remains little evidence that it has changed practice patterns in the U.S. And while absence of evidence is not evidence of absence, the point here is precisely that an actor such as CMS has the power through reimbursement structure to create incentives and payor schemes that facilitate the move to a kind of narrative practice that could well improve the culture of pain in the U.S.

There are a dizzying number of ways and methods for implementing such a different kind of reimbursement structure into the Medicare program, but this chapter does not focus on the bowels of Medicare law and regulation, nor on its looming changes under ACA. Nevertheless, a reasonable basis exists for thinking that a reform of Medicare reimbursement policy to encourage the processes of listening to and engaging the lifeworld of the pain sufferer could have a significant impact on changing the behavior and practices of providers for the better in terms of the treatment of pain.

CMS is one actor who maintains the capacity to change the behavior of one of the intended target audiences (providers). However, it are not the only actor that possesses such power. While CMS represents the top-down means to altering practices and behavior as to the treatment of pain, a bottom-up approach is also needed to increase the likelihood of changed practices. Aristotle correctly emphasized the idea that humans are habitual creatures, and predictably, anthropologists have long pointed out that changing behavior is extraordinarily difficult. To maximize the opportunity to do so, pain policies should exert effects from multiple directions at once. If CMS is among the best-positioned stakeholders to apply top-down force to the behavior of providers in constructing the culture of pain, who or what entity is appropriately positioned to apply analogous force from the bottom-up?

Another way of asking this question is to query what forces play the most significant roles in shaping the professional practices providers will carry with them into encounters with pain sufferers. If we want to change the culture of pain, presumably a prime place to begin is by reassessing the ways in which providers are educated and learn the practices that far too often seem to at least contribute to the ubiquitous undertreatment of pain. Thus it is no surprise that many pain scholars suggest that one of the most important loci for improving the undertreatment of pain is via professional education.[27]

I agree with those pain scholars who suggest that provider education plays an important role improving the undertreatment of pain. Even trained listening is not by itself sufficient to qualify for Morris's concept of "clinically effective listening." Obviously, a certain set of technical competencies and skills are required to handle the various complexities that accompany chronic pain. Where I part ways with some of these observers, however, is in my assessment of the form such education should take. Nevertheless, because I agree that education is one of the most important means of shaping healing practices among providers, it is a suitable bottom-up approach for impacting the behavior of such providers within the culture of pain. As such, Pain Policy Recommendation #2 reads as follows:

PAIN POLICY RECOMMENDATION #2

Because education is crucial in determining providers' healing practices, administrators at medical, nursing, and allied health schools should implement programs and modules for both faculty and students whose primary objective is to cultivate tolerance for subjective knowledge.

This Recommendation requires further explanation. First, it is true that undergraduate medical students receive no instruction in pain medicine, and their exposure to the subject typically comes in the form of a single-semester course in anesthesiology, which is not equivalent to pain medicine.[28] The same generally holds true as to specific courses related to pain in nursing schools and in allied health programs. There is little dispute, then, that health professionals require far more training in the competencies and skills needed to manage effectively the wide variety of complex chronic pain syndromes and disorders.

As such, most calls to improve the culture of pain management suggest a higher priority for pain in health professional education. This is a reasonable idea, but there is reason to question how much improvement is likely to follow from granting pain elevated status in the hierarchy of health professional pedagogy. The reason for skepticism is because the conceptual schemes traced in this book promote intolerance for subjectivity and invisible pathologies like pain. Such representations deeply shape the meaning of pain in American society and are primary culprits in its undertreatment. It is therefore unclear how providing more instruction in the material causes and explanations of pain—the only explanations that fit comfortably into the biomedical model—will substantially improve the treatment of pain.

There is, however, an even deeper problem with simply adding formal courses to professional education. Namely, a solid body of evidence suggests that formal pedagogy plays only a small role in determining the healing practices of physicians.[29] In contrast, what appears to be significantly more important in shaping these practices are the "informal" and the "hidden curriculum," respectively.

In a seminal 1998 article, sociologist Frederic Hafferty argues that "a great deal of what is taught—and most of what is learned—in medical school takes place not within formal course offerings but within medicine's 'hidden curriculum.'"[30] Hafferty defines the "hidden curriculum" as a

> set of influences that function at the level of organizational structure and culture. . . . The hidden curriculum highlights the importance and impact of structural factors on the learning process. Focusing on this level and type of influence draws our attention to, among other things, the commonly held "understandings," customs, rituals, and taken-for-granted aspects of what goes on in the life-space we call medical education.[31]

In addition to the hidden curriculum, the informal curriculum is a significant component of medical education, and refers to "an unscripted, predominantly ad hoc and highly interpersonal form of teaching and learning that takes place among faculty and students."[32] The hidden and informal curricula construct some of the moral bases for the medical school community. These concepts "also challenge medical educators to acknowledge their training institutions as both cultural entities and moral communities intimately involved in constructing definitions about what is 'good' and 'bad' medicine."[33]

The idea is that if change in the practices of providers related to pain is desired, introducing a course on pain into the formal pedagogy may be unlikely to have the desired effect. If much of physicians' practices and conduct are shaped through both the informal and the hidden curricula, a pain policy recommendation should target these paradigms. As Kelly Edwards has succinctly put it, the emphasis should be on what is learned, rather than what is formally taught.[34] Hafferty suggests that the learning that occurs within the hidden and informal curricula "must be acknowledged as a legitimate source of learning, and, when necessary, countered."[35] I argue that the practices, attitudes, and beliefs towards subjective knowledge about illness experiences habituated in the hidden and informal curricula ought to be countered. I say this even acknowledging that these habits and practices are themselves reflective of deeper cultural and social narratives regarding invisible pathologies, objectivity, and pain. From a policy perspective, the idea is that countering these attitudes and beliefs as they are incorporated within the professional practices of healers is an important node for action.

The question is, to improve the undertreatment of pain, what should medical, nursing, and allied health students and teachers learn? I say "teachers" here because the basic lesson of the informal and hidden curricula is that medical students form habits in large part by modeling their behavior, habits, and attitudes from their mentors, teachers, and superiors. This is what it means to understand health professional education itself as a cultural phenomenon; habits and practices are formed in local social worlds, and primarily by and through the peer and mentoring relationships at the heart of health professional education in the U.S. Accordingly, if changing practices is the goal, it is inadequate to focus on the students, for so much of their behavior and practices are formed through modeling their mentors. Thus, one problem with the proposal to introduce pain courses in the undergraduate health professional curriculum is that it does nothing to address practices, attitudes, and beliefs of the senior educators, mentors, faculty, and administrators towards the meaning of pain.

So, what should medical, nursing, and allied health students and teachers learn? And if formal pedagogy is not the most effective means of teaching virtuous practice, how should the teachers learn? How can they be taught?

These are enormous questions that I cannot hope to resolve here. However, I can suggest a promising direction, one that is expressly mentioned in Pain Policy Recommendation #2: cultivating respect for subjective knowledge. Recall that the roots of the problem are the objectifying tendencies of the clinicopathologic method. From a health humanities perspective, then, the most promising means of improving the treatment of pain is to develop and encourage modes of clinical knowing that respect and value subjectivity and all the uncertainty and ambiguity that follows.

How can this be done? There is any number of possibilities, though some of them—like requiring practical training in the phenomenology of illness—require a fundamental reconceptualization of the goals and structure of health professional education. Other suggestions, however, do not seem to necessitate any such radical reshaping. One is as simple as encouraging admissions committees to actively seek out and even prefer applicants with humanities backgrounds over students with natural science backgrounds. The justification for this is the evidence that students with humanities backgrounds display significantly more tolerance of ambiguity than students with exclusively natural science backgrounds.[36] Dogra, Giordano, and France suggest "that selection bias toward students with such applied scientific backgrounds may contribute to a pervasive technocentrism and technophilia, and with it cognitive dissonance toward appreciating the presence and value of subjectivity and/or uncertainty in medical practice."[37] Hopefully, in this book I have disentangled at least some of the historical, social, and cultural links between technocentrism, mechanical objectivity, and intolerance for subjective, invisible phenomena in American medicine and science.

If there is merit to this view, the value of targeting for admission applicants with humanities backgrounds is nothing so amorphous as the "enhancement of educational diversity." Rather, the idea is that doing so may facilitate the development of clinical character in ways that respect and value the subjectivity of the illness sufferer. Given the significance of informal peer groups and modeling in determining healing practices, encouraging the selection and development of students more able to understand the importance of ascertaining what it is like for the patient to live in pain is all the more important.

In addition, insofar as cultural diversity education requires tolerance of subjectivity, ambiguity, and uncertainty, the methods used to teach the role of culture in health and illness may also encourage the development of providers who value subjectivity. Such cultural instruction is frequently targeted at both practicing health professionals and medical students, therefore suggesting a possible point of action for working with both mentors and trainees in cultivating a different, more virtuous culture of pain.

Dogra, Giordano, and France found that

> physicians in training wish to receive concrete information from which they can generate 'do and don't lists' for use in clinical practice . . . while students recognize that cultural diversity training is needed . . . they still expressed a strong desire for certainty-based, factual information.[38]

Such a means of teaching, however, "cannot establish the subjectivity and humanitarian appreciation that is the conduit for the medical relationship."[39] Thus, the form of instruction itself carries a great deal of weight in shaping what is meaningful about subjective, ambiguous phenomena like culture. This is exactly what Hafferty suggests is integral about the hidden curriculum. The simple act of changing cultural instruction in health professional education away from the notion of objective facts about culture and towards appreciation of the dynamic, multivalent, highly subjective ways in which cultures and subcultures inform experiences of illness may have a positive impact in changing attitudes, practices, and beliefs towards the highly subjective phenomenon of pain.

These suggestions—increasing recruitment of students with a humanities background and altering the method of instruction as to the role of culture in experiences of health and illness—are simply two examples of ways of cultivating greater respect for subjective knowledge as to illness experiences into the education of professional healers.

These first two Pain Policy Recommendations reflect a two-pronged approach to one of the three target audiences identified in response to Policy Process Question #4: providers. To change the practices, attitudes, and beliefs of providers towards the treatment of pain, recommendations were issued as to CMS (Pain Policy Recommendation #1) and as to provider education (Pain Policy Recommendation #2).

However, as I have emphasized throughout my analysis, focusing simply on health care providers is unlikely to improve the undertreatment of pain in the U.S. Providers are important, but their attitudes, practices, and beliefs as to the treatment of pain are deeply shaped by larger social and cultural factors related to the meaning of pain in American society. Pain sufferers and caregivers themselves participate in this broad discourse about pain, and that participation also shapes the attitudes, practices, and beliefs of pain sufferers and caregivers. Yet simply identifying the actors whose practices should change is insufficient; it is crucial to take the additional step of inquiring which actors or entities have the power to change pain sufferer and caregiver practices?

Question #4b: Who Has the Ability to Change the Behavior of the Target Audience? (Political Actor)

In Chapter 2 (this volume), I reviewed the evidence that the alienation pain sufferers experience from their physicians is in some ways even more devastating than that which they experience from their caregivers. This counterintuitive observation can be explained in terms of the social role physicians play in the U.S., and in the investiture that vulnerable, sometimes desperate illness sufferers make in perceiving their physician as their savior. Commentators have often referred to this as the "rescue fantasy," which is not intended as a pejorative, but as a characterization of a key device illness sufferers, caregivers, and physicians alike utilize to make meaning of illness experiences. Thus, because of the social importance physicians play in treating illness sufferers, physicians in particular and providers in general are well-positioned to alter attitudes and beliefs of pain sufferers and caregivers as to pain. Accordingly, my third Pain Policy Recommendation addresses these actors.

Question #5b: What Policy Is Recommended to Achieve the Behavior Change in the Target Audience?

> ### PAIN POLICY RECOMMENDATION #3
>
> Because pain sufferers and caregivers' attitudes, practices, and beliefs towards pain are crucial to improving its treatment, health care providers should educate pain sufferers and caregivers on the legitimacy of subjective knowledge of the body in pain.

Given my focus on centering the experiences of the pain sufferer, one immediate question is why it is necessary to educate the pain sufferer him- or herself of the legitimacy of their own subjective experiences? After all, the pain sufferer does not generally enjoy the capacity of denying their own pain experiences.

However, there is a distinction to be drawn between denying the reality that one is in pain and denying that one's pain is legitimate. One can logically accept that one is in pain but simultaneously deem such pain to be socially and culturally illegitimate. Thus, ethnographies of pain sufferers demonstrate that at times they do delegitimize their own pain and the pain of others, and that they are participants in rituals and acts that contribute to the general invalidation of subjective knowledge of the body in pain.[40] The clearest example of such a ritual is the frequency with which pain sufferers join providers in the use of diagnostic and imaging techniques, in a sometimes desperate search for visible, material pathologies and lesions that can objectify their pain.[41] The fact that pain sufferers and caregivers actively participate in such a ritual is unsurprising given the ways in which the emphasis on objectivity play such fundamental roles in constructing the meaning of illness in American society.

Acknowledging that we have much to learn from pain sufferers does not preclude the possibility that pain sufferers can learn from other participants in the culture of pain. Indeed, there is an active literature on patient education, of which a particularly important facet is the current movement towards teaching disease management to chronic illness sufferers. The available evidence suggests that the toll of suffering for many chronic diseases could be ameliorated through use of such management techniques.[42] There is little reason to think that, especially in its chronic forms, pain is an exception to these findings. In keeping with the other recommendations, Pain Policy Recommendation #3 is issued at a fairly high level of generality. Thus, it is helpful to cite some examples of what cultivating respect for subjective knowledge for pain sufferers and caregivers might consist of.

First, as noted above, one of the most common meaning-making rituals in the clinical pain encounter for both providers and pain sufferers (and presumably caregivers as well) is the use of imaging techniques in the attempt to objectify pain. This is in keeping with the general proliferation of imaging techniques in the culture of biomedicine; numerous studies have documented enormous increases in both the amount of imaging equipment in the U.S. and in the use of such equipment.

Thus, an obvious way in which providers could work with pain sufferers and caregivers to cultivate appreciation of the legitimacy of subjective experiences of pain is to suggest that clinical imaging techniques are, depending on the type of pain, unlikely to reveal anything, and, more importantly, are needed neither to legitimize the sufferer's pain *nor to treat it effectively.* The concern over treating pain in the absence of determining the underlying cause of that pain has a long history in Western medicine. Cohen notes that medieval physicians and healers were concerned with such masking. McTavish points out the same as to nineteenth century physicians: "Analgesics would only conceal the symptom, not cure the condition. Because pain usually indicated that something had gone wrong in the body, it was demonstrably foolish and harmful to mask it with drugs before its source had been determined."[43]

Nevertheless, there is good evidence that a great many pain experiences can be relieved even in the absence of a finding of visible, material pathologies. In other words, despite the powerful tendency in American medicine to link pathological anatomy with clinical reality, there is no question that people can and do experience a variety of illnesses in the absence of visible, material pathologies. In their study on the meaning of diagnostic imaging tests as to chronic back pain, Rhodes et al. conclude that

> [w]hat these patients suggest, and what studies confirm is that diagnostic imaging tests often fail to provide a solution—or even a meaningful diagnosis—for chronic back pain. Our work suggests that we might consider looking elsewhere for sources of satisfaction and meaning for these patients. One possibility might be the exploration of creative ways to develop the potentially healing gesture of 'looking at results together.'[44]

This is at the heart of Pain Policy Recommendation #3: we should consider looking away from objectifying imaging techniques in helping pain sufferers and caregivers find meaning in their lived experiences of pain, and that helping pain sufferers and caregivers do so by eschewing the automatic turn to imaging techniques is a means of cultivating respect and tolerance for the subjective, lived experiences of pain. Rhodes et al. also suggest that providers "actively engage patients' desire for agency and self authorship in the exploration of alternative solutions" as a means of assisting pain sufferers on their meaning-making journey.[45] This is an excellent example of a way of working to equip pain sufferers and caregivers with viable tools for making meaning of pain, though there are many other possibilities.

Two further points are warranted here. First, my critique here is not intended to condemn the use of imaging techniques in the treatment of clinical pain. Insofar as such techniques actually help providers diagnose and treat pain, that is all to the good. But it does not follow that the almost reflexive turn to such techniques, especially with troublesome or contested disease categories such as pain, is without economic and social cost. And one of the social costs is that the proliferation of such techniques reinforce the social and cultural frames that contribute to the delegitimation and stigma experienced by so many pain sufferers. Moreover, there is reason to believe that such imaging techniques are both not helpful in many of the clinical encounters for which they are used[46] and even greater reason to believe that imaging techniques are decidedly unhelpful in treating many kinds of chronic pain.[47] Carragee notes specifically that "MRI or radiography early in the course of an episode of low back pain do not improve clinical outcomes or reduce costs of care."[48] Similarly, a 2009 systematic review and meta-analysis of the efficacy of lumbar imaging for chronic low-back pain demonstrated the lack of any significant difference in clinical outcomes between those who received such imaging and those who did not.[49] One of the coauthors of this review, Richard Deyo, referred in a contemporaneous editorial to what he termed "imaging idolatry," and expressly connected it to the culture of pain I have described at length: "Patients are often desperate for an explanation of their pain, and visual evidence is particularly compelling."[50]

Second, the idea that providers work to cultivate in pain sufferers and caregivers greater respect and tolerance for subjective knowledge of the body in pain obviously assumes that providers have themselves cultivated such respect and tolerance. Indeed, this is precisely the subject of Pain Policy Recommendations #1 and #2. Pain Policy Recommendation #3 therefore builds off of the prior recommendations. Providers, pain sufferers, and caregivers alike are all key actors in shaping the meaning of pain, and evidence-based pain policies must address all of them.

The possibility that the constant recourse to medical imaging may exacerbate the tendency to stigmatize and invalidate the lived experiences of pain is crucial given the likelihood that pain stigma is at once common and is inequitably distributed. Three of the most obvious reasons for this stigma are

1. the fact that chronic pain typically does not present with visible material lesions that may be clinically correlated;
2. the fact that chronic pain frustrates the mind-body dualism that still exerts a tremendous effect in shaping understandings of pain among all participants in the culture of pain; and
3. the fact that pain resists quantification and measurement by the technical armamentarium available to health care providers.

Of course, there are likely many additional reasons why chronic pain stigma seems so common and so intense in the U.S., but these three factors count among the most significant explanations. Thus, any offer of ethical, evidence-based pain policy must address such stigma and seek to ameliorate it on both clinical and ethical grounds. The clinical justification for targeting chronic pain stigma through policy is the robust evidence that stigma and discrimination are bad for your health. That is, stigma is independently correlated with a number of negative health outcomes.[51] However, as Scott Burris points out, even stigma had no such adverse effects on health, it is simply pernicious in its own right and is ethically intolerable.[52]

Addressing chronic pain stigma through the first few Policy Process Questions shows the following:

Question #1: What Is the Problem? How Does It Manifest?

The problem is the stigmatization of pain sufferers, and especially the stigmatization of chronic pain sufferers. It manifests itself in the form of relatively common, intense, and persistent stigmatization of those who suffer from chronic pain. Moreover, it also manifests in inequities in the risk of being stigmatized—some subgroups seem more likely to be stigmatized than others for their pain.

Question #2: What Would Success Look Like? (Goal)

Success would look like a world in which people suffering from chronic pain were not consistently treated with skepticism and suspicion, were not marked out as different and deviant. Success would be a world in which the default is that chronic pain sufferers have their reports of pain validated and legitimized, in which their suffering was viewed with compassion and kindness rather than indifference and hostility. Finally, success would be a world in which more vulnerable and marginalized subgroups were no more likely than any other groups to experience chronic pain stigma (of equal severity).

In turning to the critical Questions #3 and #4, however, attempts to ameliorate pain stigma through policy encounter a peculiar obstacle: there is reason to believe that almost anything will work. The best example of this phenomenon is in the sustained attempts to minimize HIV/AIDS stigma, which has historically been severe across the globe. By some measures, efforts to reduce HIV/AIDS stigma have been at least somewhat successful. The authors of a 2011 systematic review note that 14 out of 19 studies reviewed demonstrated effectiveness in reducing HIV/AIDS stigma, although they also noted that only two of those 14 achieved quality ratings of "good" evidence.[53]

Thus, if interventions directed to local health care providers can work at the same time as national and global antidiscrimination efforts, it is difficult to ascertain precisely whose behavior it is that we should seek to change, and which political actors have the capacity to effect that change. Because addressing pain stigma likely requires a bundle of policies directed at all number of actors, this particular policy recommendation should be taken as merely an example of a promising pain policy.

Question #3: Whose Behavior Needs to Change in Order to Achieve the Goal? (Target Audience)

However important national and even global actors are in shaping pain stigma, public health acts and practices are inevitably local. Moreover, the social role of the physician for pain sufferers and the likelihood that health care providers in general are sources of stigma for pain sufferers provides ample justification for targeting policies intended to alleviate pain stigma at health care providers.

Question #4: Who Has the Ability to Change the Behavior of the Target Audience? (Political Actor)

Although a number of different actors enjoy the capacity to alter provider behavior, Pain Policy Recommendation #1 shows how significant a broad-based federal agency like CMS can be in signaling changes in health policy. Pain Policy Recommendation #4 targets the rules set by another federal agency, The Social Security Administration ("SSA"). SSA is critical insofar as it promulgates rules and regulations regarding the disposition of disability claims, a large number of which include reports of disability and dysfunction due to chronic pain. Legal scholars have long observed that the process for disposing of Social Security disability claims encourages suspicion, skepticism, and ultimately stigmatization towards pain sufferers. Indeed, this suspicion is literally enshrined into the Social Security Act itself.

Specifically, 20 C.F.R. § 404.1508 requires that claimants seeking Social Security benefits prove that their physical or mental impairment results

> from anatomical, physiological, or psychological abnormalities which can be shown by medically acceptable clinical and laboratory diagnostic techniques. A physical or mental impairment must be established by medical evidence consisting of signs, symptoms, and laboratory findings, not only by [the] statement of symptoms.[54]

Companion provision § 404.1528(a) explicitly declares that a patient's self-report of their own symptoms is insufficient to establish the existence of a qualifying impairment. Subsections (b) and (c) define the kinds of signs and laboratory findings, respectively, that constitute evidence of such an impairment. Psychiatric signs are allowed under subsection (b), but must be "specific psychological abnormalities, e.g., abnormalities of behavior, mood, thought, memory, orientation, development, or perception" that *must* be shown by observable facts that can be medically described and evaluated."[55]

Legal scholar Dara Purvis concludes that the strict language of the Act and its implementing regulations renders subjective self-reports of pain meaningless unless such reports can be confirmed by "objective" medical evidence.[56] The very definition of a qualifying impairment is one that can be clinically correlated with anatomical or physiological abnormalities. Psychological causes are technically accepted, but observe that such causes are the last in the grammatical series, and note further that the pathologies deemed to prove the disability must be demonstrable by acceptable clinical and laboratory techniques. This, of course, shows the dominance of the clinical gaze, the emphasis on discrete material pathologies that can be seen and objectified via the techniques of the clinic and the laboratory.

What is evident here is that the influence of mechanical objectivity and its implications for pain reaches into federal law itself. This in turn is unsurprising given the power and scope of cultures of pain. Indeed, law itself is fundamentally a discursive product, which means that attitudes, practices, and beliefs towards pain and its legitimacy shape legal regimes employed to govern it, and vice versa.

One can imagine how claims of disability resulting from chronic pain fare under this regime. Objective, medical signs and laboratory findings are required to confirm experiences of pain sufficient to trigger disability benefits under the Social Security Act. Of course, since objective signs of chronic pain are, to put it mildly, difficult to come by, it follows that the very structure of Social Security benefits engenders suspicion and skepticism if not outright stigma of those experiencing the quintessential subjective phenomena of chronic pain. Thus does the culture of pain reach into laws and policies at the highest level. Moreover, health care providers are intimately involved in the process of certifying Social Security disability claims, which means that the derogation of subjective reports of pain in the regulatory regime shaped providers' attitudes, practices, and beliefs towards pain reported by individuals in connection with disability claims.

Question #5a: What Policy Is Recommended to Achieve the Behavior Change in the Target Audience? (Ignore Perceived Limitations)

In this way, the Social Security disability benefits scheme facilitates attitudes, practices, and beliefs of suspicion and skepticism towards people claiming that their chronic pain experiences constitute an impairment for which Social Security benefits should flow. These concerns are translated into

---

PAIN POLICY RECOMMENDATION #4

Because alleviating pain stigma is critical to improving the undertreatment of pain, U.S. Congress and the Social Security Administration should amend the Social Security regime by eliminating the requirement that an individual's subjective reports of pain be corroborated by objective clinical evidence to qualify as a legitimate impairment.

Pain Policy Recommendation #4 is targeted at both the U.S. Congress and at the SSA because it is the specific statutory language in the Act that initiates the process by which subjective reports of pain are derogated. However, the SSA's rules and regulations reiterate this rank ordering, and it is therefore important to capture the entire legal and regulatory regime that serves to institutionalize and enable pain stigma. Again, this policy recommendation is merely illustrative of the kinds of policies that are needed to ameliorate the widespread yet inequitably distributed burdens of pain stigma in the U.S.

These four policy recommendations, if implemented by actors who enjoy the capacity to change behavior, justify at least a hope that such action would improve the treatment of pain. A skeptical reader could well argue in response to my policy recommendations that they are really demanding nothing short of a total culture change in order to improve the undertreatment of pain. In fact, this is no criticism at all, at least not of this particular book.

Indeed, the point of departure for this project is the observation that despite decades of intensive efforts and resources, the undertreatment of pain has not only by most reasonable metrics failed to improve, but also has arguably worsened, at least if expansion in pain-related inequities is taken as sufficient criteria of worsening. Saying as such is in no way intended as a denigration of the well-intentioned efforts so many people, organizations, and institutions have devoted to improving regard for and treatment of pain. But the uncomfortable fact of the relative ineffectiveness of those efforts remains. Throughout this book, I have argued that the most earnest efforts to improve the undertreatment of pain have had little appreciable effect in large part because they are not directed at some of the primary causes of that phenomenon in American society. And many of those primary causes turn out to be rooted in vast structural and historical edifices of Western as well as peculiarly American attitudes towards issues of pain, legitimacy, and objectivity.

David Morris is correct in arguing that understanding the American culture of pain is the key to improving its undertreatment.[57] This is in some ways unfortunate, because changing culture is arduous and protracted under the best of circumstances, and may be quite impossible in others. Nevertheless, there is no alternative. Outside of fundamental efforts to understand and reshape some of our most deeply rooted social and cultural frameworks for understanding pain, there is reason to think that even the most passionate and committed efforts to improve the undertreatment of pain will continue to produce few tangible results.

NOTES

1. Deborah Stone, *Policy Paradox: The Art of Political Decision Making,* rev. ed. (New York, NY: W. W. Norton, 2002).
2. I expressly disavow the pejorative sense of the term "rhetoric." As noted in the Introduction to Chapter 8 (this volume), rhetoric was the most significant liberal art for the humanists, at least in part because rhetoric was most able to "move men's hearts" to the cultivation of virtue, to paraphrase Petrarch. Of course, this is not to claim that rhetoric is intrinsically good—Socrates disabused this notion effectively in the *Gorgias*—but that because of the power of rhetoric to encourage virtuous practice, its capacity to facilitate virtuous health policy is ethically important.
3. This, of course, is the classic(al) notion of *decorum* in rhetoric. See Gary Remer, "Rhetoric as a Balancing of Ends: Cicero and Machiavelli," *Philosophy and Rhetoric* 42, no. 1 (2009): 1–29; Remer, *Humanism and the Rhetoric of Toleration.*
4. The EDICT Project: Policy Recommendations to Eliminate Disparities in Clinical Trials," accessed April 2, 2013, from http://lifebeyondcancer.org/edict/EDICT_Project_Booklet.pdf.
5. For an extensive discussion of the links between stigma and blame in context of chronic pain, see Daniel S. Goldberg, "Job and Stigmatization of Chronic Pain," *Perspectives in Biology & Medicine* 53, no. 3 (2010): 425–38.
6. "Social Security & Medicare Trust Fund Report," accessed October 7, 2011, from http://www.ssa.gov/OACT/TRSUM/trsummary.html.
7. CMS calculates that the ACA will add more than $575 billion to the Medicare Hospital Insurance Trust Fund during the next decade. Centers for Medicare & Medicaid Services, "Affordable Care Act Update: Implementing Medicare Cost Savings," accessed March 5, 2013, from http://www.cms.gov/apps/docs/aca-update-implementing-medicare-costs-savings.pdf. However, CMS projected in 2012 that Medicare spending will rise through 2019 regardless of the implementation of ACA; what the latter will apparently do is reduce the rate of increase, from 6.8% to 5.3% over the period. Ibid., p. 3. Hence it follows that Medicare expenditures will continue to comprise a substantial percentage of domestic GDP.
8. Jonathan Oberlander, *The Political Life of Medicare* (Chicago, IL: University of Chicago Press, 2003); Theodore R. Marmor, *The Politics of Medicare,* 2nd ed. (Hawthorne, NY: Aldine De Gruyter, 2000).
9. C.F.R. § 488.5 (2006). The Autumn 1994 (vol. 57, no. 1) issue of *Law and Contemporary Problems* is a theme issue on Joint Commission's deeming power, entitled "The Place of Private Accrediting Among the Instruments of Government."
10. Stanley B. Jones, "Medicare Influence on Private Insurance: Good or Ill?" *Health Care Financing Review* 18, no. 2 (Winter 1996): 153–61.
11. Jozien M. Bensing, Debra L. Roter, and Robert L. Hulsman, "Communication Patterns of Primary Care Physicians in the United States and the Netherlands," *Journal of General Internal Medicine* 18, no. 5 (May 2003): 335–42;

Anthony L. Suchman, Kathryn Markakis, Howard B. Beckman, and Richard Frankel, "A Model of Empathic Communication in the Medical Interview," *Journal of the American Medical Association* 277, no. 8 (February 26, 1997): 678–82; Michael Simpson, Robert Buckman, Moira Stewart, Peter Maguire, Mack Lipkin, Dennis Novack, and James Till, "Doctor-Patient Communication: The Toronto Consensus Statement," *British Medical Journal* 303, no. 6814 (November 30, 1991): 1385–7; Arthur Kleinman, *The Illness Narratives: Suffering, Healing and the Human Condition* (New York, NY: Basic Books, 1988); Brody, *Stories of Sickness.*

12. Jackson, "Stigma, Liminality, and Chronic Pain."
13. Leder, "The Experience of Pain."
14. The reason I doubt CMS causes such problems in listening is because of the evidence adduced in chapters 3–5 (this volume), which, in my view, suggests some of the deeply rooted social and cultural factors that impede listening to the illness sufferer. Such problems are well-documented in the historical record in the United States for at least a century, well before Medicare was enacted in 1965.
15. See, e.g., Robert A. Berenson and Jane Horvath, "Confronting the Barriers to Chronic Care Management in Medicare," *Health Affairs* Web Exclusive (June 2003): W3-37–W3-53, accessed June 14, 2009, from http://content. healthaffairs.org/cgi/content/abstract/hlthaff.w3.37; Oberlander, *The Political Life of Medicare*; Marmor, *The Politics of Medicare.*
16. Berenson and Horvath, "Confronting the Barriers."
17. Ibid., W37-8.
18. Edward H. Wagner, Brian T. Austin, Connie Davis, Mike Hindmarsh, Judith Schaefer, and Amy Bonomi, "Improving Chronic Illness Care: Translating Evidence Into Action," *Health Affairs* 20, no. 6 (November/December 2001): 76.
19. The website of the Dartmouth Atlas of Health Care states, "For more than 20 years, the Dartmouth Atlas Project has documented glaring variations in how medical resources are distributed and used in the United States." Accessed January 27, 2009, from http://www.dartmouthatlas.org/.
20. Christine K. Cassel, *Medicare Matters: What Geriatric Medicine Can Teach American Health Care* (Berkeley, CA: University of California Press, 2005).
21. On the history of quantification, see J. Rosser Matthews, *Quantification and the Quest for Medical Certainty* (Princeton, NJ: Princeton University Press, 1995); Porter, *Trust in Numbers;* and Richard H Shryock, "The History of Quantification in Medical Science," *Isis* 52, no. 2 (June 1961): 215–37.
22. See Morris, *Illness and Suffering in the Postmodern Age*, at 247–78.
23. Ibid., 263–4.
24. Ibid., 264.
25. Rita Charon, "A Narrative Medicine for Pain," in *Narrative, Pain, and Suffering*, eds. Daniel B. Carr, John D. Loeser, and David B. Morris (Seattle, WA: IASP Press, 2003), 37.
26. Ibid., 39–42.
27. E.g., Ben A. Rich, "The Politics of Pain: Rhetoric or Reform," *DePaul Journal of Health Care Law* 8, no. 3 (Spring 2005): 515–55; Ann L. Horgas and Karen S. Dunn, "Pain in Nursing Home Residents: Comparison of Residents' Self-Report and Nursing Assistants' Perceptions," *Journal of Gerontological Nursing* 27, no. 3 (March 2001): 44–53; Rich, "An Ethical Analysis of the Barriers to Effective Pain Management"; Doreen Oneschuk, John Hanson, and Eduardo Bruera, "An International Survey of Undergraduate Medical Education in Palliative Medicine," *Journal of Pain and Symptom*

Management 20, no. 3 (September 2000): 174–9; Bruce A. Ferrell, Betty R. Farrell, and Lynne Rivera, "Pain in Cognitively Impaired Nursing Home Patients," *Journal of Pain and Symptom Management* 10, no. 8 (November 1995): 591–8; Sidney H. Schnoll and James Finch, "Medical Education for Pain and Addiction: Making Progress Toward Answering a Need," *Journal of Law, Medicine & Ethics* 22, no. 3 (September 1994): 252–6; Morris, *The Culture of Pain.*

28. Rich, "The Politics of Pain."
29. The bulk of the literature on this matter (generally referred to as the issue of the hidden curriculum) addresses medical education. There are, however, some indications within nursing scholarship that the same dynamic affects nurses and nursing education. Katharine E. Jinks and Annette M. Ferguson, "Integrating What is Taught with What is Practised in the Nursing Curriculum: A Multi-dimensional Model," *Journal of Advanced Nursing* 20, no. 4 (October 1994): 687–95; Stephen H. Cook, "Mind the Theory/Practice Gap in Nursing," *Journal of Advanced Nursing* 16, no. 12 (December 1991): 1462–9. Reflecting the state of the evidence, much of my discussion of the hidden curriculum refers to physicians; however, unless otherwise noted, I expressly assume that the same arguments hold true for nurses and allied health professionals. Indeed, the notion of the hidden curriculum reflects a theory of education, and as such there is no inherent reason why it should not apply to healing professionals of any discipline.
30. Frederic W. Hafferty, "Beyond Curriculum Reform: Confronting Medicine's Hidden Curriculum," *Academic Medicine* 73, no. 4 (April 1998): 403.
31. Ibid., 404.
32. Ibid.
33. Ibid.
34. Kelly Fryer-Edwards, Addressing the Hidden Curriculum in Scientific Research *American Journal of Bioethics* 2, no. 4 (April 2002): 58–9.
35. Frederic W. Hafferty, "Measuring Professionalism: A Commentary," in *Measuring Medical Professionalism,* ed. David Thomas Stern (New York, NY: Oxford University Press 2006), 405.
36. Gail Geller, Ruth R. Faden, and David M. Levine, "Tolerance for Ambiguity Among Medical Students: Implications For Their Selection, Training and Practice," *Social Science & Medicine* 31, no. 5 (May 1990): 619–24; Bruce R. DeForge and Jeffrey Sobal, "Intolerance of Ambiguity in Students Entering Medical School," *Social Science & Medicine* 28, no. 8 (August 1989): 869–74.
37. Nisha Dogra, James Giordano, and Nicholas France, "Cultural Diversity Teaching and Issues of Uncertainty: The Findings of a Qualitative Study," *BMC Medical Education* 7, no. 8 (2007), accessed June 16, 2009, from http://www.biomedcentral.com/1472-6920/7/8.
38. Ibid. Among others, Linda Hunt argues persuasively that this tendency in so-called cultural competence training in medical schools is both unhelpful and counterproductive inasmuch as it signals to students and teachers alike that culture is a static, objective phenomenon containing a roster of discrete cultural truths. Linda M. Hunt, "Beyond Cultural Competence: Applying Humility to Clinical Settings," *The Park Ridge Center Bulletin* no. 24 (November/December 2001): 3–4, accessed June 15, 2009, from http://www.parkridgecenter.org/Page1882.html. Though detailed discussion of race, medicine, and culture is well beyond the scope of this project, Christian McMillen recently suggested that that this notion of culture is merely a stand-in for discredited and discriminatory concepts of race. Christian W. McMillen,

"'The Red Man and the White Plague': Rethinking Race, Tuberculosis, and American Indians, ca. 1890–1950," *Bulletin of the History of Medicine* 82, no. 3 (Fall 2008): 608–45. Moreover, this conception obviously reflects the influence of the objectifying, categorizing tendencies of the clinical gaze, in which cultural variables are parsed out into entities roughly analogous to the objective "stuff" of biomedicine.

39. Dogra, Giordano, and France, "Cultural Diversity Teaching."
40. See Chapter 2 and Chapter 5 (this volume).
41. See Chapter 5 (this volume).
42. E.g., Tanja Effing, Evelyn Monninkhof, Paul van der Valk, Gerhard Zielhuis, E. Haydn Walters, and Job J van der Palen, "Self-management Education for Patients with Chronic Obstructive Pulmonary Disease," *Cochrane Database of Systematic Reviews* 4, Art. No.: CD002990 (July 2003), doi: 10.1002/14651858.CD002990.pub2, accessed June 16, 2009, from http://dx.doi.org/10.1002/14651858.CD002990.pub2; Joshua Chodosh, Sally C. Morton, Walter Mojica, Margaret Maglione, Marika J. Suttorp, Lara Hilton, Shannon Rhodes, and Paul Shekelle, "Meta-Analysis: Chronic Disease Self-Management Programs for Older Adults," *Annals of Internal Medicine* 143, no. 6 (September 20, 2005): 427–38. Four CMS analysts recently published an article noting that evidence of cost savings and quality improvement from disease management programs for chronically ill Medicare beneficiaries is uneven at best. David M. Bott, Mary C. Kapp, Lorraine B. Johnson, and Linda M. Magno, "Disease Management for Chronically Ill Beneficiaries in Traditional Medicare," *Health Affairs* 28, no. 1 (January/February 2009): 86–98. However, Foote notes that the programs evaluated in the Bott et al. paper are extremely heterogeneous, that the primary criterion for evaluation is whether budget neutrality was obtained, and that much of the raw data for the study are either incomplete or are not publicly available. Sandra M. Foote, "Next Steps: How Can Medicare Accelerate The Pace Of Improving Chronic Care?" *Health Affairs* 28, no. 1 (January/February 2009): 99–102. Thus, judging disease management as either a failure or a success at this point seems hasty.
43. McTavish, *Pain & Profits,* 20.
44. Rhodes, McPhillips-Tangum, Markham, and Clenk, "The Power of the Visible," 1201.
45. Ibid.
46. E.g., Steven D. Pearson, Amy B. Knudsen, Roberta W. Scherer, Jed Weissberg, and G. Scott Gazelle, "Assessing The Comparative Effectiveness Of A Diagnostic Technology: CT Colonography," *Health Affairs* 27, no. 6 (November/December 2008): 1503–14.
47. See Eugene J. Carragee, "Persistent Low Back Pain," *New England Journal of Medicine* 352, no. 18 (May 5, 2005): 1891–8; Rhodes, McPhillips-Tangum, Markham, and Clenk, "The Power of the Visible," 1201.
48. Carragee, "Persistent Low Back Pain"; Fiona J. Gilbert, Adrian M. Grant, Maureen G. C. Gillan, Luke D. Vale, Marion K. Campbell, Neil W. Scott, David J. Knight, and Douglas Wardlaw, "Low Back Pain: Influence of Early MR Imaging or CT on Treatment and Outcome—Multicenter Randomized Trial," *Radiology* 231, no. 2 (May 2004): 343–51.
49. Roger Chou, Rongwei Fu, John A. Carrino, Richard A. Deyo, "Imaging Strategies for Low-Back Pain: Systematic Review and Meta-Analysis," *Lancet* 373, no. 9662 (February 7, 2009): 463–72.
50. Richard A. Deyo, "Imaging Idolatry: The Uneasy Interaction of Patient Satisfaction, Quality of Care, and Overuse," *Archives of Internal Medicine* 169, no. 10 (May 25, 2009): 922. Deyo is more correct than he realizes insofar as

the compelling nature of visual evidence of pain is a primary determinant not simply of imaging but of the undertreatment of pain itself.

51. See Scott Burris, "Disease Stigma in U.S. Public Health Law," *Journal of Law, Medicine & Ethics* 30, no. 2 (2002): 179–90.

52. Ibid.

53. Sohini Sengupta, Bahby Banks, Dan Jonas, Margaret Shandor Miles, and Giselle Corbie Smith, "HIV Interventions to Reduce HIV/AIDS Stigma: A Systematic Review," *AIDS Behavior* 15, no. 6 (2011): 1075–87.

54. 20 C.F.R. § 404.1508 (2012).

55. 20 C.F.R. § 404.1528(b) (2012).

56. Dara E. Purvis, "A Female Disease: The Unintentional Gendering of Fibromyalgia Social Security Claims," *Texas Journal of Women and the Law* 21, no. 1 (2011): 85–118. Purvis also points out that for some pain conditions that are much more prevalent among women (i.e., fibromyalgia), such proof has historically been extremely difficult to marshal, thereby demonstrating the gendered aspect to the Social Security scheme itself. (Ibid.) This too should be entirely unsurprising to readers of this book. For more on the gendered nature of pain in the modern era and some of its consequences for women in pain, see, e.g., Amy Vidali, "Hysterical Again: The Gastrointestinal Woman in Medical Discourse," *Journal of Medical Humanities* 34, no. 1 (2013): 33–57; Anne Werner and Kirsti Malterud, "It is Hard Work Behaving as a Credible Patient: Encounters Between Women with Chronic Pain and their Doctors," *Social Science & Medicine* 57, no. 8 (2003): 1409–19; Morris, *The Culture of Pain*, 103–24.

57. Morris, "An Invisible History of Pain"; Morris, *The Culture of Pain*.

Conclusion

This book began with a line from an Emily Dickinson poem: "Pain has an element of blank."[1] Now, at the close of the book, it is possible to continue with the remainder of the poem:

> Pain—has an Element of Blank—
> It cannot recollect
> When it began—or if there were
> A time when it was not—
>
> It has no Future—but itself—
> Its Infinite realms contain
> Its Past—enlightened to perceive
> New Periods—of Pain.

The poet, very likely a pain sufferer herself, provides a rich and insightful window into her own phenomenology of pain: what is it like to live in pain? First, the pain is an immensity. It is so vast, so totalizing, that it contains elements of blank. It blanks out the world; as Morris puts it, "chronic pain may expand to fill the patient's entire being."[2] Pain is also personified in the first stanza of the poem; it is not the pain sufferer that cannot recollect when it began, it is the pain itself. This resonates strongly with the personification of pain ethnographers have noted; for some pain sufferers, pain becomes a kind of a monster, an invader, the entity that renders the body grotesque, foreign and ultimately nonresponsive to the owner's demands. Again, this is the phenomenological paradox of pain. As Leder puts it, pain brings one back to a body in which one is no longer at home.[3]

The pain is so vast and so immense for the speaker that it is beyond history; it is timeless and eternal: "It cannot recollect/when it began." It was not created out of nothing ("*ex nihilo*"); accordingly it has no beginning. The pain is also beyond memory. Not only does it have no recollection of when it began, there is no memory of a time in which it did not exist: "or if there were/A day when it was not." The pain is persistent, enduring, unremitting. It has no beginning, and yet it is constant and perpetual. It has always existed, a phenomenon that obviously describes the enduring chronicity of pain experiences for many people. As chapters 1 and 2 (this volume) show, large numbers of Americans do suffer pain for relatively long periods of time, and pain sufferers themselves identify the chronicity of such pain as a critical feature of their lived experiences.

For many of these pain sufferers, there is no end in sight. Where the pain has no beginning, it also has no end: "It has no future but itself. . . ." Moreover, not only is the pain endless, it also swells to inhabit the entirety of the subject's unfolding life. There is no future that is not pain. In a 1996 study, two psychologists observed that part of the lived experience of pain is a fundamental disruption in the pain sufferer's sense of time.[4] They found in chronic pain sufferers' reports of the disruption in temporality the amalgamation of past, present, and future, linked together by experiences of persistent pain. As such, the authors found that for pain sufferers "[t]he entrapment in the now makes it difficult to cope with the future."[5] Pain's "Infinite realms" therefore contain its own past. The pain is of Infinite realms, but those realms contain the past and betoken the Future at the same time. And it is the present "entrapment" that prepares the subject of the poem to receive "New Periods of Pain." The chronic pain sufferer, in the authors' words, "creates the experience of a *'long-lasting now,'* that is a 'viscous' present, a slowly fleeting time."[6]

While there is no shortage of attention to the lived experiences of pain in the scholarly literature, the premise of this book is that such attention has been poorly translated into medical encounters for which relief of pain is sought. There is widespread agreement that this lack of attention to the pain sufferer's lived, subjective experiences is a problem; yet there are few signs of any organized and sustained policy efforts to remedy the problem. Instead, the primary policy approach to the widespread and inequitable undertreatment of pain focuses on the use of opioid analgesics, which naturally centers the gatekeepers of such medications—physicians.

This book has canvassed many of the other problems with the dominance of the opioid policy approach. The idea is not that the discussion on the safe and effective use of opioids should be abandoned, but that there are profound empirical, clinical, and conceptual reasons to doubt that such a pathway is the most promising avenue to ameliorating the devastating undertreatment of pain in the U.S. The fact that safe and effective treatments exist that are sufficient to manage a large majority of the pain experiences most Americans have suggests the problem is one of translation. But the translational problems are not barriers of "translational medicine" in the narrow sense of the term. The efficacy of health interventions of any kind is profoundly influenced by social, cultural, economic, legal, and political factors, which is why anthropologists continue to study the social lives of medicines and other treatments. The related idea at the core of this book is that unless one begins to understand the social and cultural factors that shape the meaning of pain in American society—which is not equivalent to those factors that shape the meaning of opioids—it is impossible to comprehend why pain is so poorly and so inequitably treated, and why pain sufferers seem to endure such persistent stigma.

As to the meaning of pain, there is too another sense in which pain has an element of blank: it is invisible to the clinical gaze. It is a blank; even acute pain cannot be captured via objective medical and scientific tools, and chronic pain is basically defined by the lack of visible lesions that could account for the pain. This invisibility has roots in nineteenth-century concepts of objectivity. These concepts still shape contemporary American understandings of pain in powerful ways, and show exactly why illness experiences that do not present with visible pathologies that can be clinically correlated pose such enormous problems in American cultures of medicine and science. But cultures of medicine and science are in turn part of larger cultures of pain, a critical point that shows an additional reason why the focus on opioids is misguided: there are many kinds of people and communities participating in the culture of pain, from physicians and health care providers to pain sufferers, caregivers, law enforcement officials, and policymakers. Ideas about objectivity and subjectivity permeate exchanges among and between all of these parties. If these ideas are primary factors in the undertreatment and stigmatization of pain in the U.S. today, it stands to reason that remedies of any kind must address them to stand any chance at creating a more virtuous culture of pain.

Changing culture is one of the most arduous tasks imaginable. William James noted that "we are all extreme conservatives."[7] The fact that James made this observation in his lecture on the meaning of pragmatism is not coincidental, for those interested in pragmatic change must grapple with this tendency to favor established habits and routines. One of the interesting questions implicated by this book's recommendations is the extent to which policy changes can alter the culture of pain, or whether cultural transformations must precede the policy changes I propose. This question is at once difficult and easy, for it is really something of a false choice. Did the 1990 enactment of the Americans with Disabilities Act reflect changed attitudes towards disability in the U.S., or did it augur, if not usher in, cultural changes that followed? Answering the question definitively seems impossible simply because of the difficulty of disentangling the myriad confounding variables to show the direction of causality. Indeed, even the attempt to discern such a direction is ill-founded given the circular, feedback-loop relationship between policy and the culture that produces it. Policies can and do shape culture, just as cultures perhaps more obviously shape particular policies.

Nevertheless, it is doubtful that public policy alone can trigger a broad-based cultural transformation. Even so, there are a number of examples in which public policies not only reflect but also catalyze and facilitate cultural changes. Although there is ample debate over the effectiveness of mid-twentieth-century U.S. civil rights policy, there is little doubt that these policy changes signaled new directions and pathways for thinking about exclusion, stigma, and discrimination in American social life. Public policy provides a starting point, one that can at least in theory have a broad effect on millions of Americans suffering pain for which safe and effective treatments exist. And at a minimum, policies can be expected to have more of an effect on behavior. Because so much behavior as to the pain of others is characterized by suspicion, skepticism, and stigmatization, using policy levers to change that behavior is an urgent ethical priority.

The pain policy recommendations provided in this book are intended to act as starting points, and there is reason to think that, if implemented, they could have a substantially positive effect. Nevertheless, there is little doubt that what I am advocating for necessitates a significant change in the culture of pain, in the way Americans interpret and understand subjective knowledge of health, illness, and their bodies. I am sympathetic to those who despair that such changes are likely or even possible. Yet I endorse them because there is no real alternative. Picking at low-hanging fruit is always attractive, especially in terms of public policy, and yet if that fruit grows remote from the roots of the problem, such efforts are virtually guaranteed to have little tangible effects.

Pain will likely always have an element of blank. But this does not imply that we lack agency to name it and to ameliorate the terrible alienation and suffering that so many people in pain report experiencing. The question, as ever, is Aristotle's: what kind of people do we wish to be?

NOTES

1. Some of the analysis that follows appears in Daniel S. Goldberg, "The Lived Experiences of Chronic Pain," *American Journal of Medicine* 125, no. 2 (2012): 736–7.
2. Morris, *Illness and Culture*, 109.
3. Leder, "The Experience of Pain," 98.
4. Christina Hellström and Sven G. Carlsson, "The Long-Standing Now: Disorganization in Subjective Time in Long-Standing Pain," *Scandinavian Journal of Psychology* 37 (1996): 416–23.
5. Ibid., 422 (emphases omitted).
6. Ibid., 422 (emphases in original).
7. William James, *Pragmatism* (1907; repr., New York: Watchmaker Publishing Co., 2010). For discussion of James's perspective specifically in context of bioethics, see Martin Benjamin, "Pragmatism and the Determination of Death," in *Pragmatic Bioethics*, ed. Glenn McGee (Cambridge, MA: The MIT Press, 2003), 193–206.

Afterword

In April 2004, I planned a weekend visit to my mother's home in Miami Beach, Florida. On the Saturday morning that I departed for Miami, Mom decided to purchase some fresh bagels for us. Having always loved the free feeling that cycling gave her, she began riding her bicycle the few blocks to the bagel shop.

She did not make it. When I walked out of the arrival gate at Miami International Airport, my younger brother Seth greeted me and informed me that Mom had been struck by a car while cycling. She did come home from the hospital later that evening, but, like many illness sufferers, her story unfolded over weeks and months. In many ways, her story is ongoing.

My father showed up after mom had laid in agony for hours on a gurney in the hallway of the hospital to which she was taken. To paraphrase Mom, my father's arrival felt like a visit from the angel of mercy. Dad is a physician, and is one of the most gentle, humane persons I have ever encountered. Naturally, I am biased in this perspective, but I have watched over the years the adoration and appreciation expressed by his hundreds if not thousands of patients. Mom and Dad divorced in 2000, but remain close friends and supporters.

Once Dad arrived, to no surprise, the pace of care picked up considerably. Yet the agony continued, not just for that day, but for months on end. Mom had suffered a fractured pelvis, which can make the slightest movement excruciatingly painful. However, the almost unendurable pain continued well beyond the expected healing time of the fracture. Mom is no shrinking violet. Ascribing to the radical feminist notion that women are people, being highly health literate, and having years of experience advocating for illness sufferers—mostly elderly persons on dying trajectories and, later, AIDS patients—as a social worker, Mom had little difficulty with assertiveness in health care encounters.

Yet, when one is in constant unending pain, it is extremely difficult to advocate for oneself. Mom needed others to advocate for her in this situation. We all tried—myself, Dad, my brother Joshua, himself a highly trained critical care and burn surgeon, and Mom's friend Marguerite, a gifted and experienced nurse and administrator. But Mom still did not get the pain control that she needed. She flitted back and forth between rehab centers, outpatient clinics, and hospitals, suffering all the while. The nadir, as both I and Mom see it, was a visit from her attending neurologist during one of her later inpatient admissions. Enraged, desperate, and weeping, Mom paged physician after physician, pleading with her providers for better pain control. While the pain medicine specialist was marginally responsive and did prescribe some of the opioid analgesics through which Mom had during those dark months achieved some semblance of relief, the attending neurologist canceled the order.

When the neurologist came to visit with Mom, a time in which she was basically beyond speech, so struck was she with pain and horror, the neurologist advised her to think 'mind over matter' and 'meditate' in lieu of opioids. After he left, Mom regained her voice long enough to inform all available providers—nurses, physicians, allied health personnel—that she was summarily firing this neurologist for his abominable behavior.

One might say in response to this occurrence that the neurologist was simply an unvirtuous, even vicious provider, and that the solution was simply to find a more sensitive, caring provider. But then, something curious occurred. Having obtained some relief from opioid analgesics, Mom requested, as best she could, that Dad or Josh help her obtain the medications. Prescribing controlled substances to an immediate family member is risky under applicable laws, but direct prescription was certainly not the only means of assisting Mom in this request, nor was it what Mom was asking for. Both Dad, who was a longtime and recognized member of the local physician's community, and Josh, who as a burn surgeon is well-acquainted with pain management modalities and interventions, certainly possessed ample resources to facilitate access to the medications through channels and pathways that had nothing to do with direct prescription. Yet, when I spoke to Dad and Josh about Mom's request, I sensed significant reluctance.

Though I am biased, if ever I fall ill, the best I could hope for with a provider would be to experience the quality of care and the humanity exemplified by Dad and Josh. So why did I sense so much reluctance, so much hesitation on the part of these gifted, highly trained, humane, virtuous healers? What could explain this?

The issues at the heart of these questions convinced me that the undertreatment of pain in the U.S. was both an important issue, and one far more complicated than the typical reasons provided (opiophobia). If even the most virtuous, most humane healers I have ever had the privilege of knowing expressed hesitation and reluctance in helping the matriarch of our family access needed and apparently effective treatments for her unspeakable and enduring pain, centering an analysis of the undertreatment of pain on the virtue or vice of the individual healer is obviously deficient. I quoted David Morris on this point earlier, but it is worth quoting again: "Blaming doctors as inhumane simply won't work." It won't work because, among other reasons, there is little convincing evidence that, whatever their collective and individual flaws, providers are any more or less humane than the rest of us, and because it is difficult to conceive that physicians are generally callous or indifferent to their patients' suffering. There is much to criticize in physician practices in the U.S., but ascribing American problems in treating pain to provider inhumanity implies a level of wantonness that is both uncorroborated and unwarranted.

So, I was convinced in 2004 and remain convinced that the reasons why pain is treated so poorly in the U.S. include but go far beyond reluctance to dispense opioids. I believed then and now that if even the best and most phenomenologically inclined physicians could display reluctance in responding to an intimate's cry for succor, the deepest and most powerful explanations for such practice had to reside in social and cultural representations of the meaning of pain. There was, I suspected, a culture of pain, and it was something about this culture and the ways in which pain is conceptualized and socialized that seemed to impede even the best and most humane providers from easing the pain sufferer's agony.

In the fall of 2005, I entered graduate school, and while I resolved to remain open on the topics and matters that most interested me, the issue of pain was never far from my mind. My mentors, colleagues, and professors have kindly indulged me in this endeavor, and this is the project that resulted, a labor of love in multiple senses.

I have, of course, purposely withheld any detailed information about the cause of Mom's pain. Does it matter? The answer is obviously 'yes' and just as obviously 'no,' depending on the dimension at issue. Ascertaining the cause of Mom's pain was certainly a useful task for a provider to engage in, but ascertaining the cause of Mom's pain was not remotely necessary to treat her far better than was done. If nothing else, readers can hopefully apprehend my suggestion that focusing on Mom's lived experiences of pain rather than the objective, discrete causes of that pain are the most promising avenue to changing the culture of pain and ameliorating its undertreatment.

Eventually, Mom did find relief, and recovered from the injuries and the trauma of her accident. But Mom now suffers from migraines and persistent low back pain, so she is still living her pain narrative. All but a very few of us either already are or one day will be doing so as well.

Index

For Product Safety Concerns and Information please contact our
EU representative GPSR@taylorandfrancis.com Taylor & Francis
Verlag GmbH, Kaufingerstraße 24, 80331 München, Germany